LIAISON PSYCHIATRY

Mental Health Problems in the General Hospital

JOAN GOMEZ, MB, FRCPsych, DPM,

Consultant Psychiatrist.
Westminster Hospital, London

CROOM HELM
London & Sydney

© 1987 Joan Gomez
Croom Helm Ltd, Provident House, Burrell Row,
Beckenham, Kent BR3 1AT
Croom Helm Australia, 44-50 Waterloo Road,
North Ryde, 2113, New South Wales

British Library Cataloguing in Publication Data

Gomez, Joan
    Liaison psychiatry: mental health
    problems in the general hospital.
    1. Psychiatric consultation
    I. Title
    616.89′1   RC455.2.C65

ISBN 0-7099-1190-4
ISBN 0-7099-1191-2 Pbk

Printed and bound in Great Britain
by Billing & Sons Limited, Worcester.

Contents

1

Overview: Scope of Liaison Psychiatry

The practice of psychiatry in a general hospital combines the factors in unfamiliar and varied settings, with an overriding intellectual challenge of identifying emotional and pathophysiological need for diplomacy. Consultation/liaison psychiatry promises to be the saviour of its parent discipline (Lipowski, 1974). It is a signpost directing psychiatry back towards the traditional medical arts at a time when it is in danger of disintegrating into a collection of social sciences (Rawnsley, 1984). In the swinging prosperity of the 1950s and 1960s, social psychiatry, community psychiatry, existential psychiatry and behavioural psychiatry all appeared. Non-medical practitioners, including social workers, medical psychologists, community nurses, nurse-therapists, marriage counsellors and bereavement counsellors, started operating autonomously, with exponents of alternative therapies abounding. A medical work-up for patients with mental disorders began to seem outmoded and intrusive, and biologically orientated psychiatrists came to be mistrusted as insensitive and mechanistic at best, and as despoilers of human rights at worst. In many countries legislation reflects this attitude, making the professional activities of psychiatrists subject to constant checking by laymen and to legal constraints. It is fortunate for the future of today's psychiatrists that liaison work has so much to offer our medical colleagues and modern students that the links between psychiatry and the rest of medicine must be strengthened by it. Collaboration is necessary for complete patient care.

It is estimated that 30 to 65 per cent of medical inpatients have significant psychiatric symptomatology, the most frequent diagnoses being depression, anxiety and organic brain syndrome, and 30 per cent of acute medical inpatients show cognitive deficits (von-Ammon Cavanaugh, 1983; Nabarro, 1984). Equally, there is a high rate of physical illness among psychiatric patients (Davies, 1965), and Granville-Grossman (1983) found 58 per cent of patients attending

1

a psychiatric clinic to have a physical disorder also. Life expectancy is reduced in depression, mania and schizophrenia, and although suicide accounts in part for the high death rate, there is also a higher than expected incidence of accident, infection and circulatory diseases. These patients are likely to come under non-psychiatric care at some time. Despite the high incidence of cognitive and emotional disorders among patients with mental and surgical disorders, only 12-28 per cent of them are evaluated by a psychiatrist (Lipowski, 1977). This is partly because psychiatric distress is not sought, and unless it is troublesome or florid, may not be noticed; or it may be regarded as a normal reaction to illness, requiring no special attention. It is also understandable that the physician or surgeon should wish to look after his own patient completely, within his own team, without advice or interference from outside. He may himself prescribe subtherapeutic doses of an anxiolytic or mild antidepressant. Patients themselves often resist the idea of seeing a psychiatrist, afraid that their symptoms will not be treated seriously, or that they are being classed as 'nutters'. The primary consultant may genuinely believe that the psychiatrist can have nothing positive to offer and is likely to upset the patient into the bargain. The big divide, however, is traditional and geographical. For many years, psychiatrists worked exclusively in mental hospitals far removed from mainstream medicine, professionally isolated. This is a recipe for mutual mistrust. Added to this, until the 1960s, psychiatric treatment involved long incarceration and a slim chance of recovery.

The development of effective treatments, mainly pharmocological, enabled psychiatrists to take their place next to other physicians. Liaison psychiatry has grown out of the inclusion of a psychiatric department in an increasing number of general hospitals during this century. The first so designated liaison service was at Albany Hospital (New York) in 1902, but now there are more than 850 such services in hospitals in the United States of America. Liaison psychiatry has now become an essential part of medical student training in Europe and America (Lipowski, 1976). Of course, both physician and patient may come to welcome the psychiatrist more warmly if he attaches himself to the medical team and attends at least some ward rounds. As early as 1929 Henry offered guidelines to the psychiatrist who wished to work with physicians (Henry, 1929). These are still valid: that careful observation is more acceptable than inspired guesswork; communication should be free of jargon; and there must be flexibility in the application of theory and the choice of therapy.

Psychosomatics — a term coined by Heinroth in 1818 — flourished from the mid-1930s through the 1960s, and gave an added impetus to liaison psychiatry. Flanders Dunbar, who wrote so persuasively about the correlation between personality and somatic symptomatology, was associated with the liaison service of the Columbia Medical Center in the 1930s. However, the lopsided approach of the psychosomatists of that period, trying to fit physical diseases to particular emotional configurations (specificity theory), involved separation of mind from body, and did not hold water in practice. This led to disillusionment among general physicians and to the decline of psychosomatics.

Liaison psychiatry is tied to no one school of thought or theory, but involves the practical application of all psychiatric knowledge, ideas and techniques where they may be helpful to physicians or surgeons in the care and understanding of their patients. The Hippocratic concept is central, that both bodily and emotional disorders follow the established laws of nature, and there is a constant interplay between the two aspects. These fundamental ideas arose from a sea of magic, philosophy and religion, remnants of which still exist today. Traditional Chinese medicine based on the opposing elements, Yin and Yang, is practised side by side with scientific medicine. Lay healers flourish in the fashionable districts of the cities of Western nations, their use alternating with that of orthodox practitioners. The early Christian ethic that disease is a matter of unforgiven sin, even to the fourth generation, is enshrined by Christian Scientists, Jehovah's Witnesses, treks to Lourdes in search of a miraculous cure, and the patient's frequent plaint 'What have I done to deserve this?' René Descartes (1650) tried to separate '*l'homme machine*', the mechanical body, from the soul-mind directing it from 'a little kernel in the brain', the pineal gland. Interestingly, recent evidence suggests that this vestigial third eye, symbolised by the *bindi* on the forehead of married Indian ladies, is the controller of the biological clocks in the hypothalamus, including those directing sexual activity. In general, however, liaison psychiatrists take the anti-reductionist stance of Francis Bacon (1605). He invited us to consider 'how, and how farre the humours and affects of the bodie do alter or work upon the mind: or againe, how and how farre the passions or apprehensions of the mind doe alter and work upon the bodie'. Certainly, our aim is to restore and enhance the sympathies and concordances between the parts of the whole that he commends, through a comprehensive biological-social-psychodynamic approach.

3

COMPOSITION OF A GENERAL HOSPITAL PSYCHIATRY SERVICE

A liaison service should ideally comprise full-time and part-time psychiatric input, with trainees led by a consultant, liaison nurses, social workers, psychologists and occupational therapists. Often it consists only of part of a junior psychiatrist's time with such access to psychological and social backup as is available to the referring agent. A skeleton service of this kind will be called upon minimally, unless the psychiatrists are exceptionally committed and able doctors.

The areas that may be covered by a liaison service include all departments in a general hospital: wards, outpatient clinics, accident and emergency department, etc. Elsewhere, psychiatric help and advice may be a regular requirement in school, university and other occupational health departments, health centres and general practice surgeries, community nursing, non-medical alcoholic and drug treatment facilities, services for the elderly and the variously handicapped, and in prisons or other institutions. The liaison psychiatrist or nurse must expect to collaborate with all categories of health-care worker. Nevertheless, the major part of liaison activity arises in response to a request from a doctor in a different specialty. His requirements are paramount. Indifference, ambivalence and overt or covert hostility, often manifest in a joking manner, may be encountered by the psychiatrist from other medical men, as from the public. Each referral is an opportunity to modify such negative attitudes (Mayou and Smith, 1986).

THE COMMONEST REASONS FOR REFERRAL

(1) Diagnostic uncertainty: usually when investigations have produced no plausible explanations for the patient's symptoms, either their presence, their persistence or their severity.
(2) The patient's complaining continues despite best surgical or medical efforts, which should have settled the problem.
(3) The patient is disturbing the ordered harmony of the ward.
(4) The staff are under strain over this patient: because of his (or her) demanding behaviour, hostility or ability to manipulate, or because they have become emotionally concerned about the patient's illness.
(5) The patient seems to have a psychiatric disorder, or has a history of such.
(6) He has hinted at suicide.

4

(7)   He has nowhere to go and/or does not seem competent to manage on his own.

(8)   He has asked to see a psychiatrist.

The liaison psychiatrist has no all-embracing explanatory theory for disease and emotional upset, and no panacea.

WHAT THE LIAISON PSYCHIATRIST CAN AND SHOULD DO

(1)   Consider seriously and objectively the problem he (or she) has been invited to address and make clear, practical recommendations about this, even if these are negative or involve no change of management.

(2)   Appraise the social, biological and psychological factors producing, enhancing or maintaining the patient's symptoms.

(3)   Evaluate the extent to which the social and psychodynanic aspects contribute to the current position, including, for instance, such life events as recent redundancy and its meaning to the individual patient.

(4)   Assess the patient's personality and current psychological state, and his likely response to hazardous, uncomfortable or expensive investigations, for instance coronary angiography, or medical or surgical treatments which inevitably carry some risk of side-effects or worse.

(5)   Assess and suggest treatment for any functional psychiatric disorder arising in the course of physical illness, or already present.

(5)   Give practical advice about the care of substance abusers who are admitted to general hospital beds.

(7)   Assess and give guidance about the management of psychiatric disorders presenting with physical symptoms, for instance an anxiety state manifesting in precordial pain.

(8)   Collaborate in the management of psychosomatic illness including, among others, Alexander's 'Big Seven': peptic ulcer, bronchial asthma, ulcerative colitis, rheumatoid arthritis, essential hypertension, neurodermatitis, and thyrotoxicosis.

(9)   Diagnose and advise on the management of organic brain syndromes, giving short and longer-term prognoses: as in alcoholic and other drug-related psychoses, including iatrogenic (e.g. levodopa psychosis) and psychological manifestations of organic disease (e.g. neurological, ineffective, malignant, endocrine).

(10) Assess the causes and likely outcome of confusional states in the elderly, and make long-term recommendations, with indications as to how these may be achieved.

(11) Advise on the management of unexpectedly severe or intractable pain.

(12) Directly or indirectly provide care and comfort for the dying and their relatives. (Also staff support: see 24.)

(13) Assess suicidal risk in overdose patients and others, with recommendations on management, immediate and to follow.

(14) Educate and help patients and staff in coping with chronic disease and disability, including the psychosocial aspects, for instance in epilepsy.

(15) Support patients and advise ward staff with anxious, depressed or histrionic patients, for instance a woman with a lump in the breast awaiting surgery.

(16) Advise on the management of abnormal illness behaviour, for instance malignant hypochondriasis.

(17) Apply or advise on special techniques, for instance hypnotherapy for smoking, biofeedback for migrainous headaches.

(18) Mediate and interpret between the primary team and a hostile, mistrustful, demanding patient or his relatives.

(19) Mediate within the multidisciplinary therapeutic team.

(20) Facilitate for patients' self-understanding and avoidance of habitual maladapative attempts at coping, train in self-regulation, and try to enhance personal growth.

(21) Set up groups where appropriate, for instance for those with bronchial asthma.

(22) Teaching: education of patients, relatives, paramedical, nursing and medical staff and students in the principles of caring for the patient's whole person, and the psychiatric aspects relevant in particular circumstances, for instance that depression may be expected in acromegaly.

(23) Clinical research: many joint (psychiatric/medical) studies have been made, for instance with breast cancer, hyperventilation, bereavement and morbidity rates.

(24) Support and guidance for nursing, medical and paramedical staff, with group discussions where feasible, particularly in intensive therapy, oncology, haemodialysis and paediatric departments.

Every patient responds emotionally in some way to physical illness and to the invitation to regress implicit in medical and nursing care. The reaction depends upon the type and severity of the physical illness, its meaning to the patient and the degree to which it may disrupt his way of life. It may be seen as a threat, humiliation, punishment or perhaps a blessed relief, or reward. Frustrated physicians and surgeons, when a patient's symptoms persist, may be quick to suspect 'hysterical overlay', conversion symptoms or frank malingering. None is so well equipped to sort out the possibilities as the liaison psychiatrist, nor to recognise as soon as possible the Munchausen patient, with propensity to lead surgical colleagues in particular into interventions which are regretted.

Psychiatric patients with a known history are usually referred promptly and anxiously, sometimes with good reason: for instance, in the case of a young schizophrenic admitted to an orthopaedic ward after jumping from a third-floor window 'because the grass was green'. An urgent task for the psychiatrist is to check that the patient's psychotropic medication is compatible with what the physicians are giving: monoamine oxidase inhibitors are an obvious risk area. It is equally important to ensure that the patient continues to receive any maintenance medication, particularly antipsychotic, while he is in a general ward. Dosage may need to be increased temporarily to protect the patient from the extra stresses resulting from physical problems. Unlike neurotic patients, however, a schizophrenic patient usually stands up very well to physical illness, and complains less than other people. I know of a recent coronary bypass patient with severe chronic schizophrenia who felt no pain postoperatively and had to be reminded to stay in bed because he felt, immediately, so well.

Another group of patients who may require particular psychological monitoring themselves and whose professional therapists may also require support are the victims of catastrophe, for instance from bombing. It is important for a staff group to feel that, even when a patient has died or is deteriorating, the care they are giving is worth while, and that something can be learned from the experience, both for themselves and for the benefit of patients, present and future.

The psychological effects of physical illness sometimes amount to a clinical psychiatric disorder. They fall into four categories:

(1) Incontrovertibly organic effects, for instance an acute brain syndrome following, especially, cardiac surgery (postcardiotomy delirium).

(2) Understandable emotional reactions, but severe enough to be incapacitating, for instance depression, anxiety states, and obsessional neurosis.
(3) Those somewhere between the two, for instance, the irritability of patients with thyrotoxicosis or depression following infective hepatitis.
(4) Exacerbation or precipitation of an acute episode in ongoing functional psychosis: schizophrenia, manic depression.

Other areas of concern to the psychiatrist are the post-traumatic syndrome which may follow not only accidents and injuries received out of hospital, but also surgery which has proved disappointing in some way. Physical and psychological aspects require teasing out, usually in a setting of hypochondriasis. Psychosomatic disorders by definition require a joint approach by psychiatrist and physician, and often a rearrangement of the patient's lifestyle, in conjunction with his family or employer.

BACKGROUND THEORIES

In the late nineteenth century scientific progress made it seem probable that specific bacteria produced specific diseases, although even the great Henry Maudsley believed that 'immoral' habits such as masturbation could also induce punishing effects, for instance blindness (Maudsley, 1871). Cannon (1920-1939) studied the adaptive physiological response to emergency situations likely to require 'fight or flight'. He suggested that emotions of fear or anger followed the physiological changes, rather than vice versa. There is evidence in Schachter's work for this somewhat unlikely theory of bodily changes producing emotional states. In this research, men were induced to believe that a particular girl was more attractive than any other in a group by a simulated feedback of their own heart rate increasing when they looked at her photograph (Schachter and Singer, 1963). Selye's all-encompassing stress theory suggested that autonomic responses to danger could be triggered inappropriately and that this false firing might become habitual, with physical ill-effects, such as peptic ulcer (Selye, 1974). Wolff and his colleagues envisaged stress-induced disorders as having a symbolic meaning, for instance colonic disturbances where there is a covert desire to be rid of somebody (Wolff, 1953). From family and life histories Flanders Dunbar (1954) paired personality profiles with particular illnesses. Her impression that compulsive workaholics are the likeliest to suffer myocardial infarction is echoed in Friedman and Rosenman's (1971) current hypothesis about Type A personalities, who work compulsively, constantly under self-induced pressure of time.

In contrast to Dunbar, Franz Alexander (1950) investigated the relationships between seven recognised psychosomatic disorders and specific situations of emotional conflict. In peptic ulcer, for example, he postulated conflicting desires for dependence — being fed by others — and shame and guilt at not presenting as capable and self-reliant. Mirsky's prospective study of Army recruits (Mirsky, 1958) showed that soldiers with high serum pepsinogen levels tended to have the infantile traits described by Alexander, and that those who later developed ulcers all came from the high pepsinogen group. Mirsky's work was important in introducing a biological factor into psychosomatic disorder, which made it more understandable that psychoanalytic techniques aimed at modifying personality traits had disappointing results in psychosomatics. Engel (1980) and Parkes and Brown (1972) have demonstrated increased morbidity and mortality among the bereaved. Psychoimunology is a relevant area of research, since immunocompetence protects from infection and cancers at least. Bartrop *et al.* (1977) found bereaved spouses had depressed lymphocyte function five weeks after their loss. Green (1978) and his colleagues found that people who had undergone stressful life changes had decreased lymphocyte responsiveness. Today, the possibility of opportunist disease in those with the HTLV III (acquired immune deficiency) syndrome must be remembered.

Epidemiological studies of life events and their sequelae lends support to these studies. Holmes and Rahe (1967) developed a system of life-change units: the greater the amount of adjustment required recently, the likelier the onset of illness. Paykel (1978), working along similar lines, divided life events into exits and entrances: the former were more potent in making the patient susceptible to physical or psychological illness. Psychosocial vulnerability factors have been studied by Brown and Harris, in particular in Camberwell, London, in their book *Social Origins of Depression* (1978). These include, for women, having three or more children under the age of 14 at home, the lack of a confiding relationship, and loss of mother before the age of 11, or of a father in the middle classes before the age of 17.

Overload of the interlinked biological, psychological and sociological system complex disturbs the peripheral, autonomic and central nervous systems, including emotional state, and endocrine and immunological responses. For example, a man who had been

9

sensitised by earlier losses responded to his son's death in a road traffic accident by anger and despair, drinking too much, gastritis and unreliability at work. He lost his job, and within a few months developed a cancer. His friends felt that he had been extremely unlucky having three unfortunate events one on top of the other. The liaison psychiatrist can see a logical thread linking the parts of this patient's story.

Whereas some people respond to losses and disaster by overt emotional upset, others keep a braver front and may develop physical disorders. Nemiah (1976) postulates a condition he calls alexithymia, in which the patient is constitutionally unable to express his feelings. This is a further factor in the development of physical disorders in emotionally upset people.

The attempt to make sense of illness and disaster, and from there to work out ways in which the patient may be helped, is an exciting and fascinating task, the essence of general hospital psychiatry.

TECHNIQUES AVAILABLE TO THE LIAISON PSYCHIATRIST

(See also Chapters 14 and 15.)

Psychotropic medication is a simple and convenient line of attack, both for those who somatise their emotional problems and those who respond to their physical difficulties with psychological distress, and those who are responding by an organic brain syndrome to organic insult.

Electroconvulsive therapy can be used in dire circumstances, when rapid change is urgently needed, in actively suicidal patients, those who steadfastly refuse to eat for whatever reason, and in the severely depressed.

Removal to a psychiatric facility may be desirable, but is not always immediately feasible if the patient has, for instance, just had cardiac surgery, or needs an operation urgently.

Psychotherapy, usually brief and supportive, is helpful to the neurotically distressed in particular, with special reference to the alexithymic patient who needs help and guidance to be able to verbalise emotional matters. Group, couples and more interpretive individual psychotherapy is usually more convenient for outpatients, because of the prolonged timescale required. It may be run by non-medical professionals, preferably under supervision.

Hypnosis and autohypnotic techniques are useful, for instance in asthmatics; they induce muscular and mental relaxation and a suggestible state. Slow intravenous injection of diazepam or sodium amylobarbitone produces the same effect with absolute certainty.

Relaxation therapy helps those with muscular and psychological tensions and consequent abdominal, back and other pains.

Biofeedback, in which the patient is made aware of his own voluntary and autonomic responses, has been on the whole disappointing, but has a place in retraining victims of stroke and those who have suffered injuries to brain, nerves or muscle, and some sufferers from hypertension and migraine.

Meditation techniques produce the same physiological changes as are seen in hypnosis: bradycardia, lowering of blood pressure and slight slowing of the alpha rhythm in the electroencephalogram. They are helpful in hypertension and in anxiety states, but are no panacea.

Behavioural methods have been made into a new specialty: behavioural medicine. This is useful in helping to rid patients of maladaptive habits, for instance, abnormal pain behaviours, inappropriate eating and even epilepsy. Psychotics and hyperventilators are bad subjects for hypnotherapy, but the latter respond well to behavioural techniques.

THE ROLE OF OTHER PROFESSIONALS

The liaison psychiatrist would be crippled indeed without the collaboration of other disciplines.

Nursing staff

Ward nurses, who are with the patients 24 hours of the day, are the major source of objective information about a patient's functioning, mood, visitors, eating and sleeping; they are closer to the patient than any other professional, and are often used as confidantes. In inpatient treatment it is the nurses who provide human care and comfort, and it is they to whom patients turn in their moments of weakness, both physical and emotional. Nurses are essential allies in providing emotional support and are good at running supportive groups. Nurse-therapists are specifically trained in behavioural techniques, and community nurses follow the patients to their homes and hostels to bring treatment, comfort and sharp professional awareness.

Social workers

The social worker is frequently the key professional in a patient's care. Problems with finances, eating, housing in general, occupation, family loneliness, inability to cope — all fall in the social worker's ambit. These factors are often the major sources of illness-inducing strain on the patient. It is the social worker who arranges for the patient's rent to be paid, home to be looked after and benefits obtained, and when he or she goes home it is the social worker who calls up voluntary agencies and arranges for the isolated patient to have visitors to attend a day centre, with transport if necessary. When the dreaded word 'disposal' comes up, expectations are again centred on the social worker, who must find suitable accommodation for a usually unwilling old person, and persuade him or her to accept it. Social workers are excellent counsellors and may also run therapeutic groups and family sessions; their main disadvantage is that there are not enough of them. Probation officers provide similar information and aftercare services for those patients whose stresses are connected with the law, and frequently with appalling social conditions.

Occupational therapists

Occupational therapists are invaluable for the assessment of a patient's ability to function, for instance alone at home, cooking, using gas and electricity with safety, and remembering a basic shopping list. Concentration span for other work can also be measured. Those who have disabling arthritis, shortness of breath or progressive brain failure for instance may be assessed in their homes by the occupational therapist. He or she also provides training in the basic skills of living and in rewarding leisure activities.

Psychologists

Medical and clinical psychology have advanced so dramatically in the last decade that some psychiatrists fear a take-over of their own professional territory. Many research papers in the psychiatric journals today are written in part or entirely by psychologists. As experts in measurement, they express psychiatric values in numbers, which are susceptible to the statistical manipulation so highly valued by editors. The primary consultant may well prefer to call upon a sensible, 'scientific' clinical psychologist directly rather than a liaison psychiatrist, who may bring in 'woolly' emotional concepts and sex. From the psychiatrist's viewpoint it is extremely useful to have the assistance of a psychologist in diagnosis and for assessing at what level a patient is functioning intellectually, and whether this represents a fall-off. The psychologist may help in localising, to some extent, the areas of impairment; in the assessment of anxiety and depression; and in determining the relative likelihood of functional or organic psychosis. In the field of treatment, psychologists are behavioural experts *par excellence*, and usually have an admirable consistency of approach which gives behavioural techniques their best chance. Many psychologists are interested in group and other psychotherapy and perform it competently. Their expertise in vocational assessment may be of enormous value in the rehabilitation of a patient who has been ill and remains in some way handicapped.

Speech therapists and physiotherapists

Speech therapists and physiotherapists have an important role to play in helping to assess and treat patients with both physical and psychological problems.

Voluntary services and workers

Valuable help also comes from the voluntary services, in particular in keeping the patient in touch with reality.

Multidisciplinary teams are here to stay, and liaison is the watchword for the best possible patient care and pleasant and stimulating professional co-operation.

REFERENCES

Alexander, F. (1950) *Psychomatic Medicine: Its Principles and Applications*, Norton, New York

Bartrop, R.W., Luckhurst, E., Lazarus, L., Kiloh, L.G. and Penny, R. (1977) 'Suppressed Lymphatic Function after Bereavement', *Lancet, i*, 834-6

Brown, G.W. and Harris, T. (1978) *Social Origins of Depression*, Tavistock, London/Methuen, New York

Cannon, W.B. (1920) *Bodily Changes in Pain, Hunger, Fear and Rage*, Appleton, New York

—— (1919) *The Wisdom of the Body*, Norton, New York

Davies, D.W. (1965) 'Physical Illness in Psychiatric Patients' *British Journal of Psychiatry, 2* (111), 27-33

Dunbar, H.F. (1954) *Emotions and Bodily Changes*, Columbia University Press, New York

Engel, G.L. (1980) 'The Clinical Application of the Biopsychosocial Model', *American Journal of Psychiatry, 137*, 535-44

Friedman, M. and Rosenman, R.H. (1971) 'Type A Behavioural Pattern: its Association with Coronary Heart Disease', *Annals of Clinical Research, 3*, 300-12

Granville-Grossman K.L. (1983) 'Mind and Body', in Lader, M.H. (Ed.) *Handbook of Psychiatry, 2*, Cambridge University Press, Cambridge, pp. 5-13

Green, W.A. (1978) 'Psychosocial Factors and Immunity', preliminary report at the annual meeting of the American Psychosomatic Society, 31 March

Henry, G.W. (1929) 'Somer Modern Aspects of Psychiatry in General Practice', *American Journal of Psychiatry, 86*, 481-99

Holmes, T.H. and Rahe, R.H. (1967) 'The Social Readjustment Rating Scale', *Journal of Psychomatic Research, 11*, 213-18

Lipowski, Z.J. (1974) 'Consultation — Liaison Psychiatry: an Overview', *American Journal of Psychiatry, 131*, 623-30

—— (1976) 'Psychosomatic Medicine: an Overview', in Hill, O. (Ed.) *Modern Trends in Psychosomatic Medicine, 3*, Butterworths, London, pp. 1-20

—— (1977) 'Psychiatric Consultation: Concepts and Controversies', *American Journal of Psychiatry, 134*, 523-8

Maudsley, H. (1871) 'Insanity and its Treatments', *Journal of Mental Science, 17*, 311-34

Mayou, R. and Smith, E.B.O. (1986) 'Hospital Doctors' Management of Psychological Problems', *British Journal of Psychiatry, 148*, 194-7

Mirsky, I.A. (1958) 'Physiologic, Psychologic and Social Determinants in the Etiology of Duodenal Ulcer', *American Journal of Digestic Disease, 3*, 285-314

Nabarro, J. (1984) 'Unrecognized Psychiatric Illness in Medical Patients', *British Medical Journal, 284*, 635-6

Nemiah, J.C. (1976) 'Alexithymia: a View of the Psychosomatic Process', in O. Hill (Ed.) *Modern Trends in Psychosomatic Medicine, 3*, Butterworths, London

Parkes, C.M. and Brown, R.J. (1972) 'Health after Bereavement: a Controlled Study of Young Boston Widows and Widowers', *Psychosomatic Medicine, 34*, 449-61

Paykel, E.S. (1978) 'Contribution of Life Events to Causation of Psychiatric Illness', *Psychosomatic Medicine, 8* 245-53

Rawnsley, K. (1984) 'Psychiatry in Jeopardy', *British Journal of Psychiatry, 145*, 574-8

Schachter, S. and Singer, J.E. (1963) 'Cognitive Social and Physiological Determinants of Emotional States', *Psychological Review, 69*, 379-99

Selye, H. (1976) *Stress in Health and Disease*, Butterworths, London von-Ammon Cavanaugh, S, (1983) 'The Prevalence of Emotional and Cognitive Dysfunction in a General Medical Population', *General Hospital Psychiatry, 5*, 15-24

Wolff, H.G. (1953) *Stress and Disease*, Thomas, Springfield, Illinois

2

Assessment: Multidimensional Method

Assessment may fall into the crisis category, where an urgent opinion and practical on-the-spot management is required. Examples might include:

(1) The patient is threatening suicide and is in a dangerous situation, for instance on the hospital roof.
(2) He is threatening violence to someone else.
(3) He is behaving violently to property and/or persons.
(4) He is disorientated, probably hallucinated and behaving in an unpredictable manner, and is potentially a danger to himself or others.
(5) He is lying in a mute, withdrawn state, for instance in the intensive care unit.
(6) He is so completely out of touch with reality that no rational talk is possible and there is an urgent need to assess whether this is an organic or a functional disorder.

All these situations, and also parasuicide, will be dealt with later in this chapter. They are exceptional, apart from the last, but the standard liaison request may be urgent and important. Delay in responding must be minimal if psychiatry is to strengthen its reputation for usefulness. On the other hand, since the psychiatrist is often called in when colleagues are at a loss, there should be no hurry over the assessment itself.

PROTOCOL

(1) Referral requests

Read the referral request carefully and discuss the case with the physician, if possible, and the ward sister for certain, to make sure you understand what problem the primary team would like help with, and whether they have particular hopes or ideas about how this should be achieved. For instance, do they want the patient to be happier and more co-operative while they treat him, or do they want him taken off their hands? Do they want fresh light on the diagnosis, or do they merely want to share the responsibility of a difficult case?

Keep the object of the exercise constantly in mind. It is tempting to construct an excellent psychiatric formulation which may mystify — and madden — the referring consultant without focusing on what he needs.

(2) Recorded information

Read the medical notes, letters, social reports and results of investigations, the Kardex and Nursing Process records or other nursing records in detail for as far back as they are available: you may be the first doctor to have done so. Make a note of abnormalities at any stage, and any investigational omissions.

(3) First impressions

Take a glance at the patient before he knows who you are, and that you are coming to see him. The patient who complains of poor appetite may be tucking into a box of chocolates, or the one who denies any personal problems may proclaim her depression in her posture when she is off guard. If there is a visitor with the patient, try to pick up the emotional tone of their conversation.

(4) Introduction

Unless you are introduced by the nursing or medical staff, introduce yourself to the patient as a doctor, explaining that Dr X. or Mr Y., the consultant-in-charge, had asked especially for your opinion, because you have a particular interest in, say, severe and intractable pain, or breathing disorders. Of course, you are interested in other subjects as well, but at this particular time you are most concerned about this patient's problem area.

At this point, if the patient has a visitor, apologise for interrupting his visit and find out who he is. He may prefer to wait elsewhere, or to spend another five minutes with the patient and then leave. Give him the choice, and either way ask the patient if you can 'borrow' his visitor for a few minutes before he goes, as he might be able to help. It is essential that the patient's dignity be preserved and that any prejudices are put at rest. Do not volunteer the term 'psychiatrist' while a visitor is present, but explain this later.

If the patient asks with hostility whether you are a psychiatrist, agree at once, adding in the same breath that you are no ordinary psychiatrist but a doctor who works with surgeons and physicians among physically ill people. Remind the patient that such life-threatening diseases as stroke and myocardial infarction occur when the individual concerned has suffered more stress in the long or short term than he can sustain. There is no implication that in such cases, or the patient's case, the symptoms are 'all in the mind'.

You and the patient together will want to work out why he should have become ill, suffered a relapse or had an accident at this particular time. On behalf of his caring consultant, you want to make sure that there are no ongoing stressors or worries or background difficulties that might hold back healing or recovery, or cause him to become ill again when he leaves hospital. Point out that it is the bravest people who struggle on, never cracking emotionally or making a fuss, until their bodily functioning fails in some way and they have to let up. Although they may be carrying crushing burdens of responsibility, family and personal problems, disappointments, financial and other strains, such people seem to think it weak to complain until they are forced into it by physical symptoms. If the patient has a previous psychiatrist history, modify this approach by implying that you know he has a sensitive nervous system and that Mr X. or Dr Y. is concerned that this aspect should not be neglected while the physical problems are being investigated or treated.

It is mandatory in liaison practice to ensure from the outset that the patient accepts you as a sympathetic and understanding doctor who may have something to offer.

(5) Charts

Examine the patient's temperature, pulse, blood pressure and other charts, noting weight changes and bowel function, and most importantly, his medication. For instance, corticosteroids, anticholinergics, isoniazid and levodopa are of interest, as are the vast number of drugs that may cause depression, including antibiotics, antihypertensives, anticonvulsants and antineoplastics. (See Chapters 3 and 15.)

(6) Confidentiality

You want the patient to tell you what he really feels about his symptoms, his nearest and dearest, his sex life, any difficulties with the law, and his fears and hopes for the future. Apart from putting yourself across as a suitable receptacle for such precious and sensitive revelations, you must give the patient some reassurance of reasonable confidentiality. Make your bedside notes in an non-official notebook, not the patient's medical records, and point this out. This does not absolve you from making systematic and detailed notes, from which you will abstract all the pertinent information for the case notes later.

(7) Relatives' or friend's view (if available)

So as not to miss the opportunity of talking with someone who knows the patient, and who chances to be visiting him when you arrive, it is often expedient to ask for a short chat with the visitor straightaway before you have interviewed the patient. The answers you receive will gain relevance later, in the light of the patient's history. Because it will arouse resentment and suspicion in the patient if you spend much time in private with his visitor, discussion must be brief. After the preliminary politenesses, go straight into leading questions:

(a) What sort of person is the patient, e.g. a worrier, timid, drinks too much, basically happy, bottles things up?
(b) How has the patient's health been in general over the years?
(c) Any special problems that you know of, especially those the patient may be shy of mentioning?
(d) Any stresses concerning relatives, e.g. demanding elderly grandparent or son sniffing glue?
(e) Previous personal or family experience of illness or conflict: Why do you think the illness came on at this particular time?
(f) What do you think the patient most wants from life?
(g) If husband, wife or other partner: How is the sexual side going at present?

A formal meeting with a relative may need to be set up, but an off-the-cuff exchange is often quite revealing. Of course, detailed interviews with relatives or others, with the patient's permission, are not held in the patient's presence. Confidentiality is respected. The patient's account is not revealed to the relative nor vice-versa and each is reassured of this. Joint family discussions are not usually helpful in assessment, although they may be so later.

(8) Taking the history

This is the tool *par excellence* of the liaison psychiatrist, and appropriately is double pronged. To tease out the emotional from the organic components, it is a useful ploy to take two histories. The first should be medical, with meticulous dating; the second psychosocial, with particular reference to childhood and family illness and the chronology of life events. Juxtaposition of the two strands may indicate symptom-forming and vulnerability factors, learned behaviour patterns and previous responses to upset or change. The case of Mrs J. illustrates these points.

> *Case*: Mrs J., 34, had suffered from abdominal pains and persistent vomiting since Christmas, two months earlier. Barium meal and follow-through, endoscopy and a trial of ranitidine had revealed nothing specific. Mrs J. was not losing weight but was unable to go to work. Apart from rather severe dysmenorrhoea from the age of 15, which sometimes made her sick and prevented her from going to school, she had had no previous physical illness. Her parents had separated when she was 16, her father leaving for another woman. His behaviour had been erratic for the preceding year or two, and Mrs J.'s mother was often in tears. Mrs J. herself had been married for twelve years. In January her husband had changed his job, and since then he was often late home and seemed 'different', less warm. In fact, Mrs J. was reliving the period when her father had been breaking away from the family, and her bodily pattern was similar to what it had been then, and similarly had kept her in the spurious safety of home. In the event, Mr J. was preoccupied by complexities of his new job, which he had taken in order to earn more for his family, and he had no thought of abandoning them. His concern when his wife developed physical symptoms reassured her, and her symptoms subsided when their communications failure was repaired.

HISTORY, PART I: MEDICAL

Current symptoms

Their time and type of onset; frequency, severity; in what ways they interfere with the patient's life and activity. Precipitating, enhancing and relieving factors.

Systematic physical enquiry (see Appendix 1)

Early history: all the patient knows about his birth, mother's health in the pregnancy and after, feeding methods, and state of health as a baby. Feeding or toileting problems, if known.

School years: patient's mother's and father's health. Mother's and father's reactions, respectively, to minor illness or injury, e.g. calling the doctor; sympathy and reward; brisk and clinical approach; worry. Any illnesses, accidents or operations, chronologically, during these years.

Puberty: any physical problems; menarche; dysmenorrhoea or other problems associated with periods. Sexual orientation?

Adult life: type of work? Pregnancies or miscarriages: any problems? Births: any problems (husband present)? Previous illnesses, accidents or operations from puberty onwards, with dates and details? Anything at all similar to the current situation?

Effects of illness: how does the illness affect the patient's life? What does he or she feel about it? What do wife/husband/mother/child or friends think about it? What is the worst thing about it? Has the patient any particular fears or doubts about it? For instance, afraid it may be serious?

HISTORY, PART II: PSYCHOSOCIAL

This is the soil and setting in which the patient's symptoms arose.

Father: age, job, personality, health? (If he is dead, when, what cause, how old was the patient? Was he upset?)

Mother: as for father. How do mother and father get on together? If separated, how and when, how old was the patient, and what was the effect upon him?

Siblings: chronological order, ages, jobs, married with children, any illnesses or deaths? How does the patient get on with them, and how often does he/she see them?

Psychiatric family history

Is there anyone in the family who has been a heavy drinker, has had any nervous or psychiatric problems, or any of the psychosomatic illnesses? Make it easy for the patient to tell you of any psychiatric family history by hinting that only the dullest families have no eccentrics in them. Details of any psychiatric illnesses, diagnoses and treatment are important.

Personal history

Where was the patient born, and where was he brought up? Was he a happy-go-lucky or sensitive child?

School: did he enjoy it? What were the best and worst parts of school? How old was the patient when he left? Ask about examinations only if the patient was at school long enough reasonably to have taken them. Ask about problems with authority, and whether he had many friends, a handful, one or two, or was a loner.

What did the patient do next? Leave this open-ended to cover further education, scrappy jobs or staying at home, doing very little.

Jobs: longest lasting? Relationship with colleagues and with superiors?

Current situation and plans?

22

Psycho-sexual history

How old was the patient when he first had girlfriends or boyfriends? How old for first sexual intercourse? Important men or women in the patient's life, including the current situation.

Marriage: At what age? How old is the partner? How long had they known each other? What is the partner's job? How does the sexual side of the marriage go — in the past, and in the present? How is the patient's sexual interest in general, i.e. does it cheer him/her up to see an attractive man or woman? What is the relationship with the in-laws like? Is it on the whole a happy marriage, remembering that all women (men) can be irritating? What is the worst characteristic of the patient's partner?

Children: ages, sex, problems.

Social/financial aspects

Does the patient live in a flat or a house? Is it satisfactory; how long has he/she been there, what are the neighbours like; has the patient any money worries? When did the patient last have a holiday, and what did he do? Does the patient smoke? How much daily? Over how many years? If not, how long ago did he stop? (See Chapter 6.)

Does the patient drink alcohol? Every day? How often otherwise? What type of drink, and the maximum intake in 24 hours? Ever any problems because of alcohol? (See Chapters 7 and 9.)

Does the patient play cards or gamble *regularly*?

PAST PSYCHIATRIC HISTORY

Any psychiatric or nervous problem: as a child; as an adolescent; since becoming an adult? Any inpatient treatment — dates, type of illness, and treatment? Any outpatient or GP consultation for emotional problems (with dates, etc.)?

Women only: does the patient have premenstrual tension or depression? Has she had 'after-baby blues' or more serious postnatal illness?

What does the patient hope for in the next five years? —

occupationally, materially, in his personal life? What is his worst fear? What is the best thing that has happened in his life?

Personality

How would the patient describe himself? Add to this what you will have picked up from hearing the patient's long account of himself. Note how well or otherwise he is able to describe emotions (see Appendix 4).

Current mental state

Ask how the patient feels in his spirits, and then specifically about features of depression: i.e. poor appetite and weight loss, inability to enjoy anything, middle insomnia and early waking, diurnal variation of mood, lethargy, feelings of guilt and low self-esteem, constipation, retardation, agitation and poor concentration.

Ask about features of anxiety or tension: tachycardia, tremor, frequency of micturition and perhaps of bowel action, sweating, poor concentration, restlessness, initial insomnia, ready fatigue, and inability to cope. If a patient denies depression or anxiety, yet has some of the characteristic features, consider a diagnosis of masked depression or masked tension. Patients who have physical symptoms frequently pour all their emotional problems into these physical symptoms with a relief, comparatively, of the emotional side.

Check through Appendix 2, or if you suspect an organic problem, check through Appendix 3.

SUPPLEMENTARY PHYSICAL EXAMINATION

Although you do not wish to repeat examinations that have been made by the original team, it is a mistake to believe that colleagues are infallible, even in their own field. If there is any doubt in your mind, having read the previous records, repeat them. This is particularly important in neurological cases, and the psychiatrist should be prepared to do a neurological examination (see Chapter 5). To feel the pulse or to try the plantar reflexes is non-intrusive, and sometimes extremely valuable, even if nothing more extensive is done.

OPINION AND RECORD IN THE MEDICAL NOTES

Since psychiatry deals in 'soft' data, a clear concise written opinion is vital. It should comprise:

(a) *Points from the history*: these supplement where relevant what has already been elicited and recorded by the referring team.
(b) *Impression*: probable psychiatric diagnosis, with supporting evidence, with differential diagnosis, and assessment of the patient's basic personality. The contribution of the psychological factors to the physical symptoms, and vice versa, and the patient's likely response to treatment, should be delineated.
(c) *Recommendations*: further investigations, drug treatment with dosage, timing, desired and possible side-effects; other treatments and future management. Care must constantly be taken to use plain words and understandable concepts. Suggestions for such measures as long-term psychotherapy should not be made without the ability to implement them.

It is important for the psychiatrist to make it clear when he has nothing to offer: it is all too tempting to suggest something simply because one has been asked as a last resort.

To clarify complex information, a grid may be useful (see Table 2.1).

Table 2.1: Patient Evaluation Grid. Modified from Leigh and Reiser, 1980.

Factors	Current	Recent	Background
Environmental (social)			
Behavioural			
Psychological			
Biological			

SPECIAL SITUATIONS

The patient is in a dangerous situation, threatening suicide

It is essential to develop a dialogue between the patient and one person, who should preferably be situated in the direction of safety, for instance inside rather than out on a balcony. The person speaking to the patient should remain in the same place once he has made verbal contact with the patient, at least while the situation is sized up. Meanwhile, safety measures may quietly and discreetly be arranged, for instance fire-service ladders and rescue gear, and extra staff out of sight inside the building. If the patient is in a high and dangerous place and becomes frightened, it is better to reassure him and tell him to stay quietly just where he is until help comes to him, rather than to risk his, or anyone else's, safety climbing along a ledge prematurely.

If the patient has a sharp instrument and threatens to kill himself, continuous talking is more effective than trying to 'rush' him. Try to lead the discussion into areas other than the current situation, either talking about bland areas such as his birthday, where he lives, where he was born, or what he wants to do if everything goes well for him, and he receives sufficient help. Once he has agreed to part with his weapon or come into a safer place, the same person who has been talking with him should stay with him, continuing the discussion. If the setting is in a hospital, the patient should be persuaded and helped to go to bed, and given sedating medication by any route: diazepam, if this is judged to be a neurotic upset, or chlorpromazine if a psychotic element is suspected. The patient will usually accept a cup of tea meanwhile. If the incident occurs other than in a hospital, the patient must travel, escorted, in an ambulance to hospital; he may need sedation on the way.

The patient is threatening violence to somebody else

Again, the most important response is to establish a dialogue with the patient and to get the intended victim to move to a safer distance as soon as possible. When there are enough back-up staff, they should guide the patient from both sides to a separate room and sedate him with intravenous or intramuscular haloperidol:

26

probably 30-50 mg will be required. In the US it is more usual to give 5-10 mg every hour until the desired degree of sedation is required (Lipowski, 1980). Procyclidine 10 mg may also be given by the same route. The patient will have a dry mouth and be glad of a drink of tea while the medication takes effect.

The patient is behaving violently to property and/or people

In this case, the patient is past the point of listening to or even hearing what anyone is saying, and although it is sensible to try talking with him initially, it will only be a time filler while sufficient help is assembled effectively and safely to control the patient physically. Again, intramuscular or intravenous haloperidol (30-50 mg) or droperidol (10 mg) is relatively safe for the cardiovascular system and in epilepsy. They do not have too prolonged an effect if diagnosis is unclear. Give procyclidine 10 mg if necessary. In the US smaller (10 mg) repeated doses of haloperidol are used: see above. Droperidol, although categorised as a 'neuroleptic (tranquillizer) agent in the *Physicians' Desk Reference* (1986) is not specifically recommended in psychiatric emergencies.

The patient is disorientated and probably hallucinated, behaving in an unpredictable manner, potentially dangerous to himself or others

A brief history is essential in this circumstance. For instance:

Has the patient had an injury? If so, did it involve the head?
Could there have been much blood loss internally or otherwise?
Does he smell of alcohol?
Is there any knowledge or indication of illegal drug use, for instance needle tracks?
Any possibility of organic solvents?
Has he had a fit, or is he a known epileptic?
Any evidence of cardiorespiratory disease? Is he on medication, such as anticholinergics, antihistamines, or has he had previous anaesthesia?
Any reason to suspect cerebral secondaries?
Any indication of infection?

27

A fluctuating course, worsening in the evening and at night, a tendency to misidentify unfamiliar people and objects as familiar ones, and — if available as an emergency — a diffuse slowing of the electroencephalogram indicates an organic as opposed to a functional psychosis or hysterical dissociation.

If organicity seems likely, a full neurological and medical examination and investigations are urgently needed; head injury or subarachnoid haemorrhage in particular must be excluded.

As a holding manoeuvre while results are awaited and the patient is acutely disturbed, the safesty drug to use is haloperidol. (See Appendix 3 and Chapter 5 for further information.)

The patient is mute and apparently inaccessible

The pressing problem is to distinguish an organic from a functional disorder. A detailed neurological examination is an urgent necessity (see Chapter 5), as is assessment of the level of conscious awareness. The term 'mutism' implies that the patient is conscious.

Is the patient drowsy but rousable? Does he drift back into sleep? What type of stimulus is needed to elicit a response, for instance quietly saying his name, giving a simple command, shaking or painful stimuli followed by a command?

What kind of response results? Verbal, motor, appropriate or uncoordinated?

Does he appear to understand speech, shown by his responses, even if mute?

Differential diagnoses to consider include neurological syndromes, such as the 'locked-in syndrome', and akinetic mutism. In the former, a lesion at the level of the pons produces quadriplegia and mutism, with full consciousness and the ability to communicate by moving the eyes and eyelids. In the second condition it is the reticular formation which is damaged, and the patient, although apparently aware of his surroundings, is inaccessible. Neurological signs will be found in each of these syndromes. Post-ictal stupor is a temporary effect which may appear as mutism, and the neuroleptic malignant syndrome is an iatrogenic condition, usually occurring in young men, with rigidity, hyperthermia and pallor. Remember also severe motor dysphasia, dysarthria and haemodialysis 'dementia'. Functional disorders which may produce mutism are retarded depression, catatonic schizophrenia, and hysterical conversion. If a functional disorder is suspected, it is worth talking to the patient about someone with whom he is emotionally concerned, or making reassuring or stimulating statements while counting the patient's pulse rate. Variations when sensitive topics are mentioned indicate a large psychiatric component. In such cases, a conversation in whispers may sometimes be induced.

Occasionally, in the intensive care unit a patient may remain markedly unresponsive and mute although his blood chemistry and other investigations are normal. In such cases intramuscular injections of clomipramine 25 mg once or twice, may start off the return to obvious awareness and responding.

The patient is so completely out of touch with reality that no rational talk is possible

An acute organic brain syndrome may be associated with infection, trauma, space-occupying lesion, vascular disorders, epileptic, toxic, endocrine or metabolic disorders, cardiorespiratory disease leading to hypoxia, and vitamin deficiency. The same grouping, with the addition of degenerative diseases, also applies for chronic organic syndromes. Most of these disorders are considered in detail in the systematic (Chapters 5 to 13). Organic possibilities must always be considered before making a functional psychiatric diagnosis. A high index of suspicion of organicity, at any rate in part, is important, and Weir Michell's dictum (1890, quoted in Trimble, 1981) should be remembered: 'the symptoms of real disease are painted on an hysterical background'. On the other hand, response to every situation, including that of physical disease or the fear of physical disease, is influenced by the patient's personality, beliefs about the causation of illness, his interpersonal relationships and the meaning and importance of the symptoms to him.

Deliberate self-harm and parasuicide

A large number of patients are admitted each year, especially in certain urban areas, because of deliberate self-harm. Methods range from overdosage, by far the commonest, to jumping from high buildings, or cutting the wrist or neck. Whereas physicians and surgeons will deal with the immediate practical aspects, it is the psychiatrist who must find out why the patient took such action, what was his state of mind then and now, and — most importantly — whether he poses a serious, ongoing suicidal risk. In this context it is important to remember that most people, especially after an overdose of anti-depressants, have a temporary lift of spirits during their admission; that the apparent dangerousness of a suicidal attempt has little relation to the patient's intentions; and even those patients who patently did not intend to die this time stand a 4 per cent risk of killing themselves during the next year. A full history is essential for what is a commonplace to the doctor, but a major event to the patient. There is a large healing element in being allowed to tell an attentive listener the whole story, and the background.

Deliberate self-harmers fall into several categories:

(a)   those whose life situation makes them feel miserable, tense and helpless, often because of a failed relationship. They want everything to stop, at any rate temporarily, and hope for some change later;

(b)   those who are depressed and in despair, perhaps as part of a manic-depressive illness, or because of a severe loss such as major bereavement;

(c)   those who are physically ill and wish to avoid further suffering, or becoming a burden to others;

(d)   those who wish to manipulate parents or partners, or to escape the law;

(e)   psychotic patients, either schizophrenic or suffering from paranoid depression, who believe for delusional reasons that they should die or injure themselves.

All patients need care, but some need guarding against their suicidal propensities.

Assessment of suicidal risk.

Loading factors include:

(a)   male sex;

(b)   elderly but not very aged;

(c)   physical ill-health;

(d)   violent method, for instance, hanging, jumping, shooting (cutting wrists is usually merely an expression of tension);

(e)   history of depressive or manic depressive illness;

(f)   history of having prepared for death by updating the will, or

      giving away property;
(g)   delusional state;
(h)   intense humiliation;
(i)   lack of emotional support.

If there are several risk factors, the patient requires careful observation and removal to a psychiatric ward as soon as this is feasible.

APPENDIX 1: SYSTEMATIC PHYSICAL ENQUIRY

Do you have a cough? ....   With sputum? ....
Do you wheeze? ....
Sinus trouble? ....
Night sweats? ....
Pain in the chest? ....
Short of breath? ....
Palpitations? ....
Ankle swelling? ....
Varicose veins? ....
Difficulty in swallowing? ....
Nausea? ....
Vomiting? ....
Heartburn? ....
Indigestion? ....
Flatulence? ....
Pain in the abdomen? ....
Constipation? ....
Diarrhoea? ....
Easy bruising? ....
Rash? ....
Sore tongue? ....
Headaches? ....
Dizziness? ....   Sense of rotation? ....
Fits? ....
Faints? ....
Unsteady walk? ....
Pins and needles, or numbness? ....
Weak? ....
Difficulties with sight? ....
Ever see double? ....
Deaf? ....

Difficulty with passing water?.............................

Frequency of passing water?.............................

Pain in joints?.......................................

Stiff joints? ....

Swollen joints? ....

Pain in back? ....

Sore eyes? ....

Itching? ....

Very thirsty? ....

Cannot stand the heat?............   The cold?............

Sweating too much? ....

Tremor?...

Neck swelling? ....

Pain with periods? ....

Irregular periods? ....

Premenstrual tension?................................

Any other physical problems? ....

....

Tobacco: How much?   How long?

Alcohol: How often?   Maximum in 24 hours?

Medicines?

Other drugs, e.g. ginseng, cannabis?

APPENDIX 2: MENTAL STATE EXAMINATION

Tick or underline where possible.

Patient's Name _____   Date _____

Appearance:	Dress: Neat/Untidy/Abnormal/Clean/Dirty
Self-care:	Good/Indifferent/Neglected
Behaviour:	Co-operative/Friendly/Hostile/Suspicious/Retarded/
	Normal/Overactive/Fidgety/Relaxed/Tense/
	Distractible/Tremor/Stereotyped movements/Tics
Speech:	Spontaneous/Only in response/Pressured/Slow/
	Fast/Mute/Coherent/Incoherent/Circumstantial/
	Perseveration/Word salad/Neologisms
Mood:	Depressed/Anxious/Cheerful/Elated/Angry/
	Withdrawn

Affect: Appropriate/Incongruous/Blunted/Labile
Thought: *Content*: Delusions/Misinterpretations/Over-valued ideas/Phobias/Obsessional thoughts/Ideas of reference/Passivity experiences/Insertion/Blocking/ Broadcasting/Confabulation
Form: Flight of ideas/Poverty of thought/Concrete thinking/Formal thought disorder

Perceptual Disorders

Hallucinations: Auditory: Voices talking to patient/About patient/Thought echo/Other sounds/ Functional hallucinations
Visual: Olfactory/Tactile/Gustatory/ Autoscopy/Misidentification.

Cognitive State: Place/Month/Year/Time of
Orientation: day/Person

Concentration: Months backwards/Serial sevens time taken and mistakes)
Conceptual- isation: Proverbs: Concrete/Normal/No idea
Memory: Short term: News; Name and address to recall later
Long term: World War I; World War II — dates
Insight: Good/Bad/Indifferent
Intelligence: Previous — from achievements; Current

APPENDIX 3: MENTAL STATE EXAMINATION FOR ORGANIC BRAIN SYNDROMES

1. *Consciousness*
   clear
   clouded
   fluctuant
2. *Affect*
   apathetic
   euphoric

    paranoid

    anxious

    normal

3. *Hallucinations* (ask for as dreams, or of other people behaving oddly or badly.) Visual/auditory; when occurring: day/evening/night.

4. Ask the patient to remember a flower, food, colour, town; tell him to think of a flower and tell you what it is — for instance, daffodil, then food, and so on. (See point 14.)

5. *Orientation*: what building is this; the name of the ward; where is your home? how do you get there? day, month, year; which meal comes next? age and date of birth; who is looking after you here?

6. *Mental arithmetic*: ask the patient to double threes (normally, people easily get up to 1,536; stopping before 192 shows a functional intelligence quotient of 20 or less).

7. *Brief paired associates test*: teach the patient that if you say 'east' he must say 'west'; if you say 'hand', he must say 'foot'; if you say 'king', he must say 'queen', and then repeat them in a different order, giving only the first word; then do a different group: cup/plate, cat/milk, gold/lead. Any faults bring the patient into the dementia range.

8. *Meaning of a proverb* that the patient has heard of.

9. *News*: current and long past, for instance, who was Winston Churchill? where did the Beatles come from?

10. *Digit span*: start with three only, forwards and backwards. Normal would be seven forwards, six backwards.

11. *Visuo-spatial facility*: show the patient a circle drawn on paper and ask him to put the numbers in to make a clock, and, if he does this efficiently, to put in the hands showing, for instance, the time of ten to four. Ask the patient to draw a bicycle, and to copy a shape you have drawn, for instance a diamond or star.

12. *Test for nominal aphasia*, remembering that it is the details such as the teeth of a comb, the hands of a watch, the buckle of a shoe, that cause difficulty.

13. *Test for tactile agnosia*: ask the patient to close his eyes and identify objects put first into one hand and then the other, for instance, a pen, a coin, a ring, a piece of paper, a closed safety pin.

14. Ask the patient if he remembers the flower, food, colour and town that he was asked to remember. (See point 4.)

15. *Perseveration*: Record whether the patient gives an answer appropriate to the previous question before he can change his mental set.

16. If the patient has not been very successful, get him to say what comes next: Our Father which art in . . ., or Jack and Jill went up the . . . .

17. *Remember* the frontal lobe syndrome: empty euphoria, incontinence, poor gait, sometimes a grasp reflex.

Remember not to alarm or humiliate the patient. Whatever answer he gives, appear pleased or a catastrophic reaction may occur.

APPENDIX 4: VERBAL EXPRESSION OF EMOTION

The questions to be asked include the following.

When someone has made you angry do you:

(a) Tell him plainly?
(b) Cry or hit out?
(c) Go away?
(d) Get a headache or other bodily feeling?
(e) Think about it a lot?

When you feel an affectionate interest in or are attracted by someone, do you:

(a) Tell the person how you feel?
(b) Talk about other subjects?
(c) Give the person a present?
(d) Think about him/her a lot?
(e) Do nothing?

How would you or did you propose or accept marriage?

(a) Explicitly
(b) Casually
(c) By implication

Did you enjoy it? Say how you felt?

How would you feel in these circumstances?

(a) Only child killed by a car

(b)   Large fortune comes your way
(c)   You are asked to be chairman of, say, neighbourhood group
(d)   You find your best friend has been robbing you
(e)   You see an old man being mugged.

REFERENCES AND FURTHER READING

Abbott, R.J. and Loizou, L.A. (1986) 'Neuroleptic Malignant Syndrome', *British Journal of Psychiatry, 148*, 47-51

Fenn, H.H. and Ochitill, H. (1984) 'An Overview of General Psychiatry', in Goldman, H.H. (Ed.) *Review of General Psychiatry*, Lange Medical Publications, California

Howells, J.G. (1982) *Integral Clinical Investigations*, Macmillan, London

Leigh, H. and Reiser, M.F. (1980) *The Patient: Biological, Psychological and Social Dimensions of Medical Practice*, Plenum, New York

Lipowski, Z.J. (1980) *Delirium: Acute Brain Failure in Man*, Thomas, Springfield, Illinois

Lishman, W.A. (1978) *Organic Psychiatry*, Blackwell, Oxford

Roberts, J.K.A. (1984) *Differential Diagnosis in Neuropsychiatry*, John Wiley, Chichester and New York

Trimble, M. (1981) *Neuropsychiatry*, John Wiley, Chichester and New York

3

Psychological Presentation in Various Disorders

The whole range of psychiatric symptomatology may present, and is relevant, in general hospital psychiatry (Sensky, 1986). To every appreciable physical symptom or sign, from a headache or a wart to crushing pain or paralysis, there is some emotional response (Mechanic, 1986). This is reflected in the temporary rise in neuroticism scores on the Eysenck Personality Inventory (Eysenck and Eysenck, 1964) that are usual among medical and surgical inpatients. Minor anxiety or depression is common currency, and frank mental illness is no rarity in association with physical disorders. The interrelationship is complex:

(1) Physical symptoms may be the presenting symptoms of an emotional disorder, for example the well known 'Monday morning' abdominal pain that afflicts the unwilling schoolchild.
(2) Emotional states with matching lifestyle may induce psychosomatic responses, for example duodenal ulcer in the stressed city bus driver, or myocardial ischaemia in the Type A business executive.
(3) Drugs, legal or otherwise, may produce subtle effects on the hypothalamic and limbic structures, or gross toxic effects in the brain, for example alcohol, diazepam, benzhexol, heroin.
(4) Trauma may produce equally dramatic effects through structural damage, or through psychological mechanisms, or there may be an interplay between the two, for example variations of the post-traumatic syndrome.
(5) In organic disease, structural, endocrine or metabolic mechanisms may influence the mental state, for example in hypothyroidism, diabetes mellitus and hydrocephalus.
(6) Toxic effects of every type may induce an overt organic brain syndrome, or, less obviously, organic irritability or lethargy, with for example, ergotamine, carbamazepine or lithium.

(7) Pain and its perception, involve mysterious two-way mechanisms, for example the excruciating pain of a phantom limb, lasting for years in a vulnerable, obsessional personality, and by contrast, the apparent absence of pain felt by a farm worker who carried his severed arm for over a mile under his other arm when he went to get help.

PSYCHOLOGICAL PRESENTATIONS OF ILLNESS

The psychological presentations of illness comprise the following: anxiety, including phobic anxiety and obsessional fears; depression, either neurotic, psychotic or pseudo-depression; hydrochondriasis; mania and euphoria; hallucinations and delusions; acute, subacute and chronic organic brain syndromes.

ANXIETY

This may be either a symptom or a response. It is a common reaction to any disorder, depending on its meaning to the patient. The panic when a newly observed mole is thought to be a malignant melanoma is a transient experience among many medical students. Unexpected difficulty in remembering a familiar name can similarly affect an older person fearing the onset of brain failure. A stiff knee for a footballer may mean missing a vital match, a career opportunity lost. A lump in the breast may mean not only a threat to health, but a threat to a failing marriage. Such anxiety is more or less consciously understood. In stroke, impending respiratory failure, before as well as after myocardial infarction, or in early dementia, symptoms of anxiety may be prominent although the patient is not aware of the cause.

The manifestations of anxiety are many and diverse, and represent autonomic overactivity, either mainly sympathetic, mainly parasympathetic, or both. They include tremor, muscular tension producing pain and stiffness, and headache; 'butterflies' in the stomach, nausea, and abdominal pains; tachycardia and raised blood pressure, palpitations and chest pain, including pain in the left arm; dry mouth, difficulty in swallowing, frequency of micturition, diarrhoea, disturbed menses, and weight loss with or without anorexia; sweating, especially in the palms and feet; and the more obviously psychological symptoms of subjective fear, irritability, restlessness, initial insomnia, and poor concentration. Hyperventilation, either episodic or a persistent habit, is an anxiety symptom that may lead to numerous secondary problems which are discussed in detail in Chapter 6. These and other anxiety symptoms may be misinterpreted as indicative of serious organic disorder, for instance heart disease or cancer. A vicious circle may be set up.

If the liaison psychiatrist can suggest some better management than the standard dulling doses of diazepam prescribed by physicians and surgeons, he will save much time and suffering. Even those patients who have organic disease as well as an anxiety state will respond better to treatment when the situation is clarified by removal of the anxiety symptoms. Busy doctors and nurses tend to feel guilty — that they are not working hard — if they take time fully to discuss, explain and reassure their patients. The value of such efforts should be emphasised although too much reassurance, or too many people giving different versions, can be counterproductive. They believe that this is wasting time unless instructed otherwise. The psychiatrist may find his own time well spent on relaxation therapy, teaching autohypnotic techniques, and desensitisation for specific fears, particularly those associated with investigative procedures and surgery (see Chapter 16).

Medication

Benzodiazepine anxiolytics such as diazepam and lorazepam have an obvious place. The former is particularly useful when muscular relaxation is desired, but has disadvantages given parenterally. With intramuscular administration, absorption is variable and much of the drug precipitates in the tissues; intravenously its irritating properties lead to thromboses. Lorazepam is generally useful dissolved and absorbed through the buccal mucosa: it is tasteless and does not have the disadvantages of diazepam by either of the parenteral routes. Dosage of 2 to 5 mg is appropriate for lorazepam by any route, or 10 to 20 mg of diazepam orally before potentially upsetting procedures such as endoscopy.

For inpatients who are continuously anxious, it is reasonable in the short term, for instance in the days running up to surgery, to give diazepam 5-10 mg b.d. and o.n., or lorazepam, 1-2.5 mg t.d.s. and o.n. The latter has a short action and needs to be given more frequently than diazepam. For the initial insomnia of anxiety, temazepam, 20-40 mg is rapidly absorbed and rapidly cleared from the system, but lormetazepam, 1-2 mg or flurazepam 15-30 mg, may be better for those anxious patients who wake on and off through the night. Lometazepam may not yet be available in the US: it has a convenient eight-hour half-life. All the benzodiazepines are mildly depressant, both to mood and to respiratory function. Some patients, particularly those with a paranoid edge to their anxiety, respond better to small doses of trifluoperazine (1 mg one to three times daily), haloperidol (1.5 mg, one to three times daily) or thioridazine (10-50 mg, three or four times in 24 hours).

For those whose anxiety is already laced with depression, sedating antidepressants may be the best choice, especially for sleep, for instance doxepin, 50 mg, trimipramine 50 mg, or lofepramine 70 mg at night. (Lofepramine, a tricyclic with minimal anticholinergic effects, may not yet be available in the US.) Beta-blockers such as propranolol and atenolol are useful in cases in which tachycardia is the most prominent feature, but are disappointing in general. Dosages of 10 to 40 mg of propranolol are suitable for anxiety symptoms. Further consideration of pharmacological aspects of anxiety is made in Chapter 15.

A mood of anxiety or even stark fear is frequently found in incipient delirium tremens and other withdrawal states, and as part of any organic brain syndrome (see below). Appropriate treatment is required for these cases even more than for disorders that may masquerade as anxiety states, for instance hypoglycaemia, hyperthyroidism and, rarely, phaeochromocytoma (see Chapter 9). Occasionally physiological, disease- or drug-induced tremor may be mistaken for the tremor of anxiety. Agitation, in which psychomotor restlessness is a key feature, may present in hypothyroidism, and as a part of agitated depression considered below.

Obsessional symptoms

Checking and endlessly repeating actions, or silently going over and over the same unwanted thought, may be an expression of anxiety. It is often released by depression and recovers as the latter lifts. Hypochondriacal thoughts are particularly common, with the patient convinced of malignancy, or, if that is a fact, of widespread metastases and early death. Apart from 'the big C' (cancer), heart disease, herpes genitalis, and, among homosexual men, AIDS are common hypochondriacal preoccupations. Reassurance loses its value if often repeated, but should be given firmly and the accompanying depression should be treated with clomipramine 75-200 mg daily, or an MAOI such as phenelzine 30-60 mg daily. Thought stopping, perhaps assisted by snapping an elastic band on the wrist to help interrupt the obsessional thought lines, is also useful.

Phobic symptoms

These may attach to investigation or treatment that is desirable, and are an expression of anxiety that requires urgent management. Again, treatment of accompanying depression should be given with the drugs useful for obsessional symptoms: the tricyclic antidepressant clomipramine, or the MAOI, phenelzine. In the short term and in emergency, lorazepam is readily absorbed from the mouth or may be given intramuscularly or intravenously; it has a short half-life of four hours. Diazepam is less satisfactory in that it has disadvantages given parenterally and is absorbed rather more slowly by mouth. However, it has a longer-lasting effect and marked muscle relaxant properties. Thioridazine is calming and sedating.

DEPRESSION

This is particularly important in liaison practice, partly because it is significantly often the harbinger of organic disease from breast cancer to hepatic failure or Alzheimer's disease. There is evidence that some forms of malignant disease, for instance lung cancer, reveal themselves after bereavement, and depressive symptoms may be the first indication of anything going wrong. Depression follows the onset of various organic illnesses. However a physical disorder has arisen, recovery is likely to be quicker and smoother if the patient is content: in childbirth, after abdominal surgery or stroke, or when the patient is battling with severe respiratory infection.

Depression embraces numerous variants on the theme of lowered mood and vitality, and cognitive impairment. It may be divided broadly into primary and secondary groups. In either group the syndrome may be mainly 'reactive' or mainly 'endogenous' in type. Reactive or neurotic depression is the commoner and is loaded with anxiety, restlessness, initial insomnia and outwardly directed blame, while responsiveness to reassurance and environmental change is retained. The 'endogenous' cluster of symptoms is most likely to arise in patients who have had previous severe depressive illness or a family history of affective disorder. The symptoms include middle and delayed insomnia, profound loss of appetite and weight loss at an alarming rate. The patient feels empty and unreal rather than low, blames himself, can make no decision and sees no hope. Such patients pose a suicidal risk, particularly if they harbour depressive delusions, for instance of their internal organs having rotted away, or of destitution. Whitlock (1982) in his monograph on symptomatic affective disorders guides us through largely uncharted waters. Symptomatic depression equates with depression secondary to physical disease or certain drugs but is by no means synonymous with reactive depression. The prognosis improves when physical disorder recedes. Much depressive illness not considered secondary to organic disease follows a cluster of unfavourable life events of which physical illness is regarded as one such. Mitchell-Heggs (1971) found 40 out of 200 depressed patients had suffered a physical illness within the previous two months. Pollitt (1971) implies that depression is precipitated rather than caused by physical illness: a matter of 'brought-forward' time theory. Klerman (1975) by contrast stresses the potential research significance of secondary depression involving, for instance, endocrine disorder. Drug-related depression may also illuminate the pathology of the disorder. Medication which may be associated with depression covers a wide range from antifungals to antihypertensives.

Drugs that may cause depression

Drugs that may lead to depression include:

Psychotropic drugs
phenothiazines, e.g. chlorpromazine
butyrophenones, e.g. haloperidol
thioxanthenes, e.g. flupenthixol (in the UK), thiathixene (in the US)
benzodiazepines, e.g. diazepam
chlormethiazole
hypnotics in general, e.g. dichloralphenazone
alcohol, as in 'boozer's gloom'
Appetite suppressants, especially fenfluramine
Cardiovascular drugs
beta-adrenoceptor blockers, especially those that cross the blood/brain barrier easily, e.g. propranolol
alpha-adrenergic blockers, e.g. bethanidine, guanethidine
alpha-adrenoceptor blockers, e.g. prazosin
central hypotensives, e.g. clonidine, reserpine

methyldopa, hydralazine
digoxin
Steroids and hormones, e.g. prednisolone, oral contraceptives, oestrogens, progestogens, cyproterone, clomiphene
Analgesics and anti-inflammatory drugs, e.g. opiates, indomethacin, ibuprofen, naproxen
Antihistamines, e.g. chlorpheniramine, promethazine
Neurological drugs
anticonvulsants, e.g. phenytoin, phenobarbitone
anti-parkinsonians, e.g. levodopa, amantidine
bromocriptine
tetrabenazine and baclofen
Antibacterials, e.g. ampicillin, tetracycline, sulphonamides, nitrofurantoin, nalidixic acid, metronidazole
Antifungals, e.g. griseofulvin, ketoconazole
Antineoplastics, e.g. vincristine, cisplatin, azathioprine
Miscellaneous
disulfiram
cimetidine, ranitidine
mebeverine
methysergide
pizotifen
salbutamol
cyproheptadine
choline

Medication which, in the constitutionally vulnerable, may precipitate severe 'endogenous' depressive symptoms includes reserpine, with 12-15 per cent incidence of depression, 5 per cent methyldopa (Granville-Grossman, 1971) and clonidine (Roberts, 1977).

The affected patients are likely to have had previous depressive episodes, although Snaith (1976), considering hypertensives, believed the severity of the disease was of more relevance than the drug treatment. With drugs such as chlorpromazine, which produce sedation, the patient's lack of sparkle and responsivity may be mistaken for depression. Sleep and appetite are enhanced rather than reduced in these circumstances.

Illnesses associated with depression

Infections, especially viral, may be followed immediately by depression. Post-influenzal, post-hepatitic, post-herpetic, post-encephalitic and post-glandular fever depression are all recognised, and measles produces misery from day one. Completed suicide is not rare in post-encephalitic parkinsonism (Slater and Roth, 1977).

Tropical infections such as malaria, sandfly fever, typhoid and dengue are frequently associated with depression. It is also reported in brucellosis and adult toxoplasmosis. In tertiary syphilis, depression is now the usual presentation (Lishman, 1978) — see Chapter 5.

The tease is: does depression reduce immunocompetence and allow an infection foothold, or vice versa?

Neurological disorders sometimes associated with depression include brain tumour, benign or malignant, in which it may be the presenting symptom. Psychiatrists need to remember this possibility which has been demonstrated at autopsy in several series (Whitlock, 1982). In multiple sclerosis, depression occurs more often than euphoria, and depression is common in Parkinson's disease and cerebrovascular disease. Depression, sometimes of suicidal intensity, may follow stroke (Adams and Hurwitz, 1974). Head injury, especially affecting the right hemisphere or the frontal lobes, is likely to precipitate depression in the vulnerable. Serotonin and dopamine levels in the cerebrospinal fluid are reduced for several months after injury (Lishman, 1978).

Storey (1972) found affective disorder following subarachnoid haemorrhage, and Trimble and Cummings (1981) described depression in patients in whom haemorrhage into the upper brainstem had disrupted adrenergic and serotoninergic neurotransmitter pathways. In Huntington's chorea there is an increased suicidal risk, and in motor neurone disease a depressive reaction is readily understandable and usual. Endocrine disorders associated with depression include hypothyroidism, hypopituitarism, pancreatic disorders, Addison's disease, acromegaly and Cushing's syndrome. Less common are hyperparathyroidism and apathetic thyrotoxicosis. Other disorders associated with depression are malignant disease of all types, hypoxia from respiratory or cardiac insufficiency, and hepatic dysfunction from whatever cause.

Pseudo-depression in organic illness is analogous to pseudo-dementia, which superficially resembles dementia. However, clinical depression is common. Table 3.1 compares the characteristics of depression and pseudo-depression.

Table 3.1: A comparison of depression and pseudo-depression

Depression	Pseudo-depression
Low mood	Mood of weariness
Lack of energy associated with 'nothing seems worth while'	Lack of energy: 'I only wish I could — but I get so tired'
Interests decline	Interests only reduced by capacity
Poor appetite	Appetite may be poor
Weight loss often	Weight loss usual
Blame directed either inwards or outwards	Vaguely apologetic for being unable to do things
Sleep disturbed	Sleep from exhaustion
Memory impaired	Memory hardly impaired

The combination of functional depression and physical disease makes for diagnostic difficulty, for instance a patient with physical illness may sleep through the night, however depressed, or be woken by pain although not suffering from clinical depression. If some of the elements of clinical depression are present, it is worth trying antidepressant therapy. Reassurance, the chance to talk and to make a relationship with one member of staff, and the cognitive approach of gradually, by reason, changing the patient's negative attitude are helpful and necessary but usually insufficient and too slow. Medication is sometimes magical and should be given. The patient who longs for a good night's sleep will appreciate a sedating tricyclic antidepressant, but for the elderly, 65 +, anticholinergic side-effects may be troublesome. These include dry mouth, constipation, urinary hesitancy, blurred vision, tremor and, in those already cerebrally compromised, confusion. In these cases a low level initiation is advisable, for instance doxepin 50 mg or trimipramine 25-50 mg at night. Pharmacological aspects are dealt with in Chapter 15, but in general amitriptyline, mianserin, doxepin, trimipramine, dothiepin and trazodone are sedating, and imipramine and viloxazine are stimulating. Maprotiline holds an intermediate position. MAOIs are useful when tension is a prominent feature, but possible drug interactions must be remembered.

HYPOCHONDRIASIS

Hypochondriasis involves a tiresome over-concern with physical health, short of the delusional except in patients with an ongoing functional psychosis. It is usually associated with depression and/or anxiety, and is particularly persistent in an obsessional personality. Treatment of depression, anxiety or obsessionality (see above) and no more reassurance than for the non-hypochondriac is the best approach. Some patients whose hypochondriasis has passed beyond the bounds of reality respond to pimozide 2-8 mg at night, and standard neuroleptic treatment is indicated for the hypochondriacal schizophrenic. He may believe that his head is square or that an infernal engine has been secretly inserted in his abdomen. Of course schizophrenic delusions may be based on an organic lesion: for instance Mr W. blamed his ischaemic leg pain on rays directed from the Chief of Police.

MANIA AND EUPHORIA

Mania and euphoria are less common than depression. Euphoria is the least common, and comprises a happy mood and feeling of well being, however inappropriate the circumstances. It is an organic response and is not usually accompanied by overactivity. Steroid medication and structural brain disease such as multiple sclerosis, general paralysis of the insane, frontal lobe tumor or Pick's disease may be responsible. Mania or hypomania includes overactivity in speech, movement and thought, with pressure of speech, flight of ideas, and a propensity to interfere. Delusions of power and importance are characteristic, running over into irritability and violence. Again, this may be precipitated by steroid medication, any of the antidepressants or bromocriptine, or it may be part of an ongoing manic depressive illness, with an episode of mania 'brought foward' in time. Cushing's syndrome and lesions affecting the right temporal lobe of the brain may induce manic symptoms. For euphoria the treatment of the cause is of major importance, whereas in mania urgent treatment, usually with haloperidol, by any route and in sufficient dosage for rapid control, is required. Untreated mania is a time bomb with a short fuse.

HALLUCINATIONS AND DELUSIONS

These are the hallmarks of psychosis, either functional as in depression, mania or schizophrenia, or organic. In general, hallucinations based on organic problems are more likely to be visual than auditory and more likely to occur after 6 p.m. unless produced by hallucinogens such as cannabis or lysergic acid. In functional psychiatric disorders, auditory hallucinations are the most frequent, usually voices. Elderly paranoid schizophrenic ladies in particular and paranoid depressives may experience tactile hallucinations, and they are also characteristic of cocaine or bromide intoxication. Phantom limb is a tactile experience usually unaccompanied by delusions. Similarly, lesions of the occipital cortex may produce complex visual hallucinations, for instance of children, but the patient is easily convinced of their unreality.

In most cases hallucinations developing in a mood of fear, common in organic mental conditions, are associated with delusions which seem to explain them. Sometimes a delusional mood leads to misinterpretation of what is perceived, and thence to frank hallucination. In this way a fearful victim of delirium tremens may see the water pipes as snakes, and deal with them accordingly. By the reverse mechanism a woman who heard hallucinatory voices plotting her destruction developed a delusional system involving the IRA, the CIA and the KGB. Delusions may arise without hallucinations rather more often in functional psychoses than organic: a schizophrenic woman believed her neighbour had buried the heads of 14 children in his garden, and a psychotic depressive man believed that he was responsible for most of the death and disease in his country. On the other hand my patient with Alzheimer's disease, aged 78, is convinced that she is 17 and wants to see her mother.

Whatever the cause, hallucinations and delusions are likely to lessen with the administration of haloperidol, and chlorpromazine also, if a longer, sedating effect is necessary. Alcoholic withdrawal symptoms do better with benzodiazepine cover (see Chapters 5 and 15), and the desperate psychotic depressive needs an antidepressant as well as his neuroleptic, and, if suicidal, urgent electroconvulsive treatment.

ORGANIC BRAIN SYNDROMES

Jaspers in 1963 pointed out that 'organic cerebral illness can occasionally show, particularly in the initial stages, every known morbid psychic phenomenon'. This remains true and makes differential diagnosis in general hospital psychiatry exciting and different. The two main organic brain syndromes are delirium and dementia, the one acute and reversible, the other chronic and often irreversible. Both are global in their effects. In fact there is a spread of gradations between these two states and in addition partial and circumscribed organic states.

Acute organic brain syndromes (delirium)

Waking and sleeping are interwoven, the sleep-wake cycle jumbled with dreams and hallucinations, thoughts and delusions intermingling. It is common as an emergence phenomenon for up to 24 hours after general anaesthesia, or lasting up to ten days postictally, in drug withdrawal or metabolic disruption. Limited cerebral reserve makes an acute brain syndrome more likely.

Causes of acute organic brain syndromes
These can be grouped into the following categories.

Toxic and metabolic: uraemia; hepatic encephalopathy; hypoglycaemia; electrolyte, calcium or magnesium disturbances; porphyria.
Nutritional: Wernicke's encephalopathy; nicotinic acid deficiency encephalopathy; hydroxocobalamin deficiency.
Infective: encephalitis; meningitis; cerebral syphilis; urinary or respiratory infection in the elderly.
Cardiorespiratory: hypoxia from cardiac or respiratory failure; embolism; hypertensive encephalopathy.
Neurological: structural lesions; head injury; subdural haematoma; subarachnoid haemorrhage; tumour; abscess; epilepsy.
Endocrine: thyroid disorders; pituitary disorders; adrenal disorders.
Drugs: alcohol and barbiturate withdrawal; acute intoxication; overdose, for example of tricyclic antidepressants; iatrogenic, for example post-anaesthetic, opiates, levodopa.

Acute organic brain syndromes come on rapidly, over a few hours. There is fluctuant impairment of attention, thought and comprehension of the environment. Electroencephalographic changes will also be fluctuant and usually involve generalised slowing.

Check for:

(1) Sun-downing: worsening of symptoms as the evening draws on
(2) Distractibility
(3) Difficulty in assessing the passage of time
(4) Disorientation in time, place and person: less common than (3)
(5) Impaired performance on, say, serial sevens, or the days backwards
(6) Hallucinations, usually visual
(7) Delusional ideas
(8) Speech slow, sparse, incoherent or shouting
(9) Movements slow, automatic, purposeless or violent
(10) Apathy *or* excitement
(11) Episodes of incontinence.

Before treatment a neurological check is necessary, particularly where there has been head injury, and it is important to know what medication or illegal drugs the patient may have ingested and to know the status of his electrolytes, urea and calcium. Any chronic systemic disease is of importance, as are anaesthetic difficulties if this is a post-anaesthetic presentation.

Management

Obvious physical problems must be dealt with, such as dehydration, blood loss or oxygen lack. The patient must not be left alone, and should be given frequent reality reminders; addressing him by name, and mentioning the time of day, the place, the next meal. Haloperidol is the most useful medication, backed up by chloropromazine or chlormethiazole if extra sedation is needed for the patient's safety. Haloperidol may be given in doses of 1.5–10 mg, repeated three to four-hourly as needed, in the elderly who are not grossly disturbed, or 20–40 mg doses for younger or excited patients. (In the US smaller doses — 5–10 mg — are repeated hourly as required, and physical restraints employed in severe circumstances.) Chlorpromazine, if needed at all, should be given in doses of 25–100 mg, also by any route. Chlormethiazole is most useful at night in oral doses of 500–1000 mg, in addition to neuroleptics by day or by day and at bedtime.

Chronic organic brain syndromes

These are long-lasting, if not necessarily permanent, and there is often progressive intellectual fall-off without such features as disorientation being obvious. Disorientation in time is the commonest. On the other hand, personality may deteriorate more than intellect, and social skills decline, or a shallowness and lability of affect may predominate. Unlike the situation in an acute organic brain syndrome, in chronic states consciousness is full. Questions about the date, including the year, the place and recent news events, should be slipped in without causing offence. (See Appendix 3, Chapter 2.)

Causes of chronic organic brain syndromes

These can be grouped into the following categories.

Degenerative: Alzheimer's disease; Pick's disease; Huntington's chorea; Creutzfeldt-Jakob disease; multiple sclerosis; Parkinson's disease; arteriosclerotic dementia.
Tumours: cerebral tumour; subdural haematoma; abscess.
Infection: general paresis (GPI); meningovascular syphilis; chronic encephalitis.
Trauma: particularly in boxers.
Endocrine: hypothyroidism; hypopituitarism; hyperparathyroidism; hypoglycaemia in diabetes mellitus.
Toxic/metabolic: alcoholic dementia; Korsakoff's psychosis; chronic barbiturate intoxication; other chemicals; uraemia; hepatic disorders.
Cardiorespiratory: hypoxia; anaemia; hypertension; congestive cardiac failure; chronic respiratory disease; post-cardiac arrest; post-anaesthetic; post-carbon monoxide poisoning.
Epilepsy: epileptic dementia.
Vitamin deficiency: lack of thiamine, nicotinic acid, hydroxocobalamin, folic acid.

A complete investigation of the possible reversible causes of dementia must be made, since management is likely to differ widely. Bulbena and Berrios (1986) describe two main types of pseudo-dementia: one associated with depression, the other with delirium. The latter is of poor prognosis for survival. Table 3.2 compares the characteristics of dementia and pseudo-dementia.

Table 3.2: A comparison of dementia and pseudo-dementia

Dementia	Pseudo-dementia
Insidious onset	Rapid onset
No previous psychiatric illness	Previous psychiatric illness
No vegetative symptoms	Vegetative symptoms
Attempts to conceal cognitive deficits	Deficits exposed
Patient tries to answer	Patient gives up
Consistently poor	Marked variability in cognitive performance
Recent memory much worse	Remote and recent memory equally poor
Sun-downing common	Sun-downing rare except in the delirious type

Of the partial and subacute organic syndromes the amnestic syndrome is common and is characterised by poor memory as the predominant clinical feature. There is no clouding of consciousness, and no general deterioration of major intellectual abilities. The memory deficit involves recent and intermediate memory and spares immediate and remote memory.

Confabulation is not a constant feature; it tends to occur early in Korsakoff's psychosis but disappears later on. Causes of the amnestic syndrome are commonly thiamine deficiency in alcoholics, cerebral trauma or any pathological process that causes bilateral damage to the mamillary bodies, fornix or hippocampal complex. Subarachnoid haemorrhage, infarction in the region of the posterior cerebral arteries, and some forms of encephalitis may do this.

REFERENCES

Adams, G.F. and Hurwitz, L.T. (1974) *Cerebrovascular Disability and the Ageing Brain*, Churchill Livingstone, Edinburgh and New York

Bulbena, A. and Berrios, G.E. (1986) 'Pseudodementia: Facts and Figures', *British Journal of Psychiatry, 148*, 87-94

Eysenck, H.J. and Eysenck, S.B.G. (1964) *Manual of the Eysenck Personality Inventory*, University of London Press, London

Granville-Grossman, K.L. (1971) *Recent Advances in Clinical Psychiatry*, Churchill Livingstone, Edinburgh and New York

Jaspers, K. (1963) *General Psychopathology*, translated by Hoenig, J. and Hamilton, M.W., Manchester University Press, Manchester

Klerman, G.L. (1975) 'Overview of Depression', in Freeman, A.M., Kaplan, H.I. and Sadock, B.J. (Eds) *Comprehensive Textbook of Psychiatry, I*, Williams and Wilkins, Baltimore

Lishman, W.A. (1978) *Organic Psychiatry*, Blackwell, Oxford

Mechanic, D. (1986) 'The Concept of Illness Behaviour: Culture, Situation and Personal Predisposition', *Psychological Medicine, 16*, 1-7

Mitchell-Heggs, N. (1971) 'Aspects of the Natural History and Clinical Presentation of Depression', *Proceedings of the Royal Society of Medicine, 64*, 1171-4

Pollitt, J. (1971) 'Aetiologocal, Clinical and Therapeutic Aspects of Depression', *Proceedings of the Royal Society of Medicine, 64*, 1175-8

Roberts, J.A. (1977) 'Dixarit (Clonidine) and Depression', *Medical Journal of Australia, 1*, 58

Sensky, T. (1986) 'The General Hospital Psychiatrist, Too Many Tasks and Too Few Roles?', *British Journal of Psychiatry, 148*, 151-8

Slater, E. and Roth, M. (1977) *Clinical Psychiatry*, Bailliere Tindall, London

Snaith, R.P. (1976) 'Hypotensive Drugs in the Treatment of Depression', *British Journal of Clinical Pharmacology, 3*, Suppl. 1, 73-4

Storey, P.B. (1972) 'Emotional Disablement before and after Subarachnoid Haemorrhage', in Ciba Symposium: *Physiology, Emotion and Psychosomatic Illness*, Elsevier, Amsterdam

Trimble, M.T. and Cummings, J.L. (1981) 'Neuropsychiatric Disturbances following Brain Stem Lesions', *British Journal of Psychiatry, 136*, 56-9

Whitlock, F.A. (1982) Chapter V in *Symptomatic Affective Disorders*, Academic Press, New York

4

Pain

Pain is at the heart of interspecialty liaison. Ninety per cent of patients presenting at medical and surgical outpatient clinics, 64 per cent of those attending generalists' surgeries, and 60 per cent of those seeing a psychiatrist complain of pain (Merskey, 1973). Such a complaint is always considered seriously. It evokes sympathy and concern from family, friends and colleagues and urgent attention from the medical profession.

Aristotle placed pain among the passions of the soul, but a more precise definition — modified Merskey — describes it as a subjective experience, involving suffering, usually interpreted as a response to tissue damage. It may sometimes be induced by disturbance in the functioning of the brain itself from overtly structural or more subtle emotional or biochemical influences. A patient's pain can only be assessed from his self-report or other actions such as groans, tears or grimaces, muscular guarding, limping or doubling up (Bond, 1979).

PHYSIOLOGICAL ASPECTS

The physiological mechanisms subserving sensations of pain are still incompletely understood. The gate control theory of Melzack and Wall (1965) accounts plausibly for many but not all pain phenomena, and lacks proof. In the simplest terms it is suggested that pain is experienced when the continuous central scanning process identifies a particular pattern of sensory input originating in small- and large-diameter afferent fibres from the peripheral nerves. The small fibres continually relay information from the periphery, but this low-level activity does not reach conscious awareness unless it is sharply increased by the local release of such intracellular chemicals as histamine, hydrochloric acid, serotonin, adenosine phosphates or potassium; or extrinsic endogenous pain-producing kinins. Modulating, sometimes inhibitory, influences are transmitted by the large-diameter fibres and central impulses impinge upon these, travelling in descending serotonergic pathways. Spicing this already subtly complex dish are the endorphins. these are relatively recently discovered morphine-like endogenous peptides found near the opiate-binding sites, and in particular abundance in the periaqueductal grey matter, hypothalamus and limbic system.

Among the neurotransmitters serotonin seems to be specifically involved in the natural pain-modifying arrangements. The administration of parachlorphenylalanine, which interferes with serotonin activity, reduces the effectiveness of morphine. Stimulation of the serotonergic nuclei of the dorsal raphe, by contrast, enhances analgesia, as does the giving of L-tryptophan, the precursor of serotonin (Cannon et al., 1978).

Acute, single-episode pain

Acute, single-episode pain is an emergency signal rushing up the large-bore rapid-transit fibres, forcing open the transmission gate, and demanding an immediate response. Overpowering inhibitory impulses occur in those exceptional circumstances in which major activity is recognised as essential to survival. In an IRA nail-bomb attack in London, six-inch nails were embedded in the tissues of the victims, mainly soldiers. None remembered registering pain as they ran from the scene in an orderly fashion, only stopping when they collapsed from loss of blood. More commonly an acute single pain is transmitted unmodified and evokes an immediate response such as screaming for help, or freezing into immobility — for instance with the pain of a perforation. The pain of myocardial infarction or renal colic tells of disaster, but is in itself dangerous if allowed to continue. Because of its harmful physiological effects it requires analgesia as soon as possible after diagnosis (Sinclair, 1973).

Chronic, recurrent or perseverating pain

Chronic, recurrent or perseverating pain is especially likely to exercise the skills of the psychiatrist in conjunction with his medical and surgical colleagues. It is this type in which non-organic influences interdigitate with the somatic, producing problems in diagnosis and management. Remaining with the physiological aspects, the summation of minor stimuli may finally overcome the inhibitory tonus and cause pain to be felt without fresh injury. The mild compression of a tight shoe may be hardly noticeable in the morning, but by evening is unbearable; with less obvious causes of mild damage a complaint of pain may be puzzling. Pain from, for instance, herpes zoster may continue long after the infection has subsided: one theory is that such pains set up reverberating circuits during the acute stage of illness, and these are slow to extinguish.

Another mechanism to account for the persistence or recurrence of pain without adequate physical cause depends on the pattern recognition process for appreciating pain. It is associated with somatic memory, which keeps particularly fresh, for instance for swimming or finding the accelerator. If part of a previous pain experience in context is detected — for instance loneliness or muscular fatigue, the whole pattern may be generated centrally. Similarly a physician may recognise a syndrome from only a few of its characteristics, sometimes inaccurately (Merskey, 1976; Trimble, 1981).

LEARNING PAIN

Pain, as already mentioned, can only be diagnosed from the patient's behaviour, audible or visible, voluntary or involuntary. Pain behaviour is learned (Tyrer, 1986).

Previous experience

Childhood exposure to pain, personal or in a key relative, may set a pattern of expectation and response. Pain, for instance from acute appendicitis, may have been invested with drama and excitement for the child, and rewarding attention from his parents. Pain may have prevented the child's attending school and brought him — or her — close to mother. Period pains are an important example. The family methods of dealing with pain and illness will colour a patient's lifelong approach to it: whether ignored as a nuisance; dealt with in a matter-of-fact fashion; responded to with sympathy, affection and new toys; or viewed as a cause for great concern and medical attention, however trivial.

The model provided by a parent or grandparent is also influential: for instance a mother who has to lie down in pain every month, getting others to do her housework, a father who is creased with pain after meals that do not suit him, or a grandmother whose arthritic pain gives her the right to be grumpy and order others about. Other maladaptive responses shown by an adult may be martyred helplessness, aggressive stoicism, ready consumption of pills or alcohol, or denigration of doctors as useless or worse (Gomez and Dally, 1977).

Operant mechanisms

Direct reinforcement is applied in the extra kindness and attention from professionals and others contingent upon the expression of pain. The elderly, who are anyway pain prone, are particularly susceptible to this reinforcer. More importantly the common practice of giving analgesics on a p.r.n. (as required) basis may act as direct reinforcement. Only when the patient indicates that he is in pain does he receive the medication. He may find not only the analgesia but also the sedation rewarding and come to request the drug in anticipation of pain that may not come at all.

Indirect reinforcement operates in the avoidance which pain permits: of arduous work, sitting an examination, sexual intercourse, a threatening social or business encounter. School students' Monday morning 'tummy aches', and socially convenient migraines are not as a rule malingering. The hope of compensation may prevent a person's returning to work and putting his pain behind him: again, seldom from a deliberate decision to deceive. Occasionally overprotective mothers, wives or husbands may discourage or even punish signs of recovery in a pain patient (Fordyce, 1978), as in the following case.

Case: Mr S.'s wife suffered from rheumatoid arthritis. During her acute attack Mr S. enjoyed cooking and a certain freedom of choice of menu. He blocked his wife's return to the kitchen by stressing how painful it had been for her handling the cooking utensils.

THE EXPRESSION OF PAIN

Most people express pain adequately but some are especially good at it: women more than men, the elderly more than younger adults, those of Jewish and Mediterranean origin compared with Scandinavians, the histrionic and extravert compared with the reserved and introverted (Harwood, 1981). Schizophrenics, who cannot easily express their feelings tend to come over as stoics. Self-mutilators, who usually have hysterical personalities, have a facility for hysterical dissociation, and feel and convey only a release of psychological tension when they cut themselves (Roy, 1982).

THE MEANING OF PAIN TO THE PATIENT

Pain may be seen as a warning or a reminder of serious disease. If the patient believes, realistically or otherwise, that he is at risk from, say, cancer or heart disease, he may become supervigilant for any hint of pain or a related symptom and report the slightest twinge or irregularity of sensation to his doctor, with a little exaggeration to ensure the latter understands its importance. Pain may be a means of communication, especially for those who find it hard to express their emotional needs: the alexithymics.

> *Case*: Mrs P.N. had three young children and an insensitive husband. She could not explain to him her need for emotional support, and developed abdominal pains which aroused both the doctor's and her husband's concern. When she recovered, her husband's interest subsided, but returned when her pains came back.

Other patients employ their pain to wield an aggressive power over others: often when an elderly parent is losing his or her sway over the family.

Pain may be interpreted as punishment by some patients: either ill-deserved, in which case they are generally resentful, or as proper retribution for their often imaginary faults. These latter are often depressives, but the need for atonement may be ameliorated by pain. Particularly in the bereaved, pain similar to that endured by the dead person may be introjected or symbolic pain may be felt: in the vagina in some widows, or in the lower abdomen after a miscarriage or termination of pregnancy.

STATE OF MIND AND PAIN

Anxiety and depression each enhance pain, and in turn chronic physical illness and chronic pain lead to depression, and in some situations such as malignant disease, anxiety. Chronic pain otherwise is not usually associated with anxiety. Irritability is common, and often resentment towards those who are well, who try to help, or who are emotionally close (Pilowsky *et al.*, 1976).

Pain is a symptom in a substantial proportion of patients with psychiatric disorders but it is found more often in neurotics than psychotics. Chronic states of emotional tension are frequently associated with pain in the neck, back, head, chest or abdomen: this is probably due to prolonged partial contraction of voluntary or involuntary muscles. Tension and reactive depression often go together but in these case stricyclic antidepressants are unhelpful, whereas small doses of anxiolytics such as diazepam may be effective in mild cases, or an MAOI in the more persistent or severe. 'Masked depression' presents with pain and manifestations of depression such as anergy, insomnia, anorexia and weight loss, but the patient smilingly denies a low mood (Lopez-Ibor, 1972). Such cases are dangerous in that suicide is not uncommon; they require close observation and prompt antidepressant measures. Other endogenously depressed patients show a delusional quality to any complaint of pain; in particular they may be convinced they have cancer and are doomed to die. Complaints of pain are not characteristic of schizophrenia, but some patients show a bizarre kind of hypochondriasis. One man felt that 'stretched biting heads' under his skin were gnawing away his body; another felt that darts were shot at him from outer space; a third believed that he had swallowed a fly in his beer some years before, causing continuous abdominal pain. Hallucinations of pain are difficult to assess since all pain is subjective and personal, but are thoeretically possible (Sternbach, 1978).

Hysterical conversion may well produce pain, but such a diagnosis, although favoured among baffled physicians and surgeons, should be made with caution by the prudent psychiatrist. Either sex may be involved, and a histrionic personality is the exception rather than the rule. *Belle indifference* is characteristic of hysterical conversion and may be manifest in apparent courage in the face of proposed surgery and a little less distress than would be expected from the patient's described pain. The patient may be highly intelligent or otherwise, but has few emotional resources.

Case: A college lecturer of 35 who still lived with his mother suffered incapacitating pain in his right arm and his legs when his college became the centre of industrial action with violent picketing. He could neither go into work nor write.

After taking a comprehensive history including previous family or personal episodes of unexplained symptoms, before a diagnosis of hysterical conversion can even be considered, plausible primary and secondary benefits must be adduced. The primary benefit is immediate escape from an unpleasant or alarming situation or threat: such as becoming pregnant for a wife under pressure from her husband, or having to leave home or do a difficult job. Although the primary fear is frequently denied, sometimes convincingly, the secondary gains are usually obvious. However, they are mainly important in maintaining symptoms already present, and may equally well apply to pains produced by physical mechanisms. Hysterical-pain patients should never be confronted with a crude diagnosis, but helped to retain their dignity while relinquishing their symptoms.

PSYCHIATRIST'S ROLE WITH PATIENTS IN PAIN

A psychiatric opinion is often requested 'to find out whether the pain is real', i.e. organic or psychogenic. In fact the best result of sifting all the information is an understanding of why this patient is suffering pain at this time, with reference to his life experience and current predicament. It is this fuller understanding that underpins psychiatric advice on how to treat the patient.

MANAGEMENT

The aim is to reduce distress, as demonstrated by the patient's behaviour, and to facilitate increased normal activity. A range of therapies is available from which to select what is most suitable for the individual. Patients with a primary psychiatric disorder should be treated accordingly; secondary depression and some anxiety are to be expected with persistent pain, and are dealt with symptomatically within the therapeutic package (Bradley, 1983).

Medication

Anxiolytics, especially those with muscle relaxant properties such as diazepam (2–10 mg, up to four times in 24 hours) sometimes ameliorate pain as well as anxiety, although they have no direct analgesic effect. They are unsuitable for long-term use since tolerance develops.

Hypnotics may be helpful to pain patients by ensuring a night's peace. Temazepam (20–40 mg) has a good initial effect; flurazepam (15–30 mg), nitrazepam (5–10 mg, not available in the US) or diazepam (10 mg) are useful in maintaining sleep.

Antidepressants: the tricyclic antidepressants, such as amitriptyline, have an inherent analgesic effect. Because of the particular role of serotonin in endogenous pain modulation, clomipramine, a serotonin agonist, is likely to be most effective. It is a drug in routine use in the hospices for terminal disease. Amitriptyline or doxepin may be more sedating, however. Of the newer antidepressants, trazodone enhances serotonin availability and is calming. Daily dosages, which may be divided or given mainly or all at night, are: clomipramine 30–150 mg; amitriptyline 30–150 mg; doxepin 50–200 mg; trazodone 50–300 mg (clomipramine may not be available in the US).

The MAOIs are the most useful in patients with chronic tension and resentment, and secondarily a neurotic depression. Phenelzine (30–90 mg divided, before 4 pm) is often the best in younger patients, whereas the middle-aged respond well to a tranylcypromine/trifluoperazine combination: Parstelin (one to four tablets daily before 4 pm). In the US the combination tablet may not be available, but tranylcypromine 10 mg with trifluoperazine 1 mg is the chemical equivalent. If MAOIs are to be used, it must be made clear to both patient and doctor that opiate analgesia cannot be used with these drugs, and they are safer stopped ten days before anaesthesia.

Neuroleptics, such as the phenothiazines and butyrophenones, have considerable pain-relieving properties, thus allowing a smaller dose of narcotic analgesics. They also reduce anxiety and counteract the confusion sometimes caused by opiates. Merskey, a leading figure in pain research, recommends pericyazine in particular (2.5–5 mg up to four times in 24 hours). Pericyazine is not readily available in the US. Perphenazine may be used similarly, in 4 mg doses.

Analgesics are basically the province of the physician or surgeon. The psychiatrist may advise on the addition or substitution of psychotropic medication in severe organic disease and benign chronic pain, respectively. In terminal painful illness, colleagues sometimes welcome reassurance about giving adequate doses of analgesia. As seen earlier, regular administration of analgesics is preferable to the 'on request' method, which encourages anticipatory reporting of pain in some patients and leaves others 'not wishing to make a fuss' by asking.

Relaxation therapy and autohypnosis may be particularly useful in patients with tension-related pain, but are also helpful in such cases as the fearful sufferer from malignant disease. After one or two sessions with the therapist the patient may be supplied with a personalised audiotape.

Hypnosis works particularly well when pain is enhanced by anxiety, and the patient is intelligent and responsive, but some alleviation may also be achieved even with pain due to serious organic damage.

Acupuncture may act either as a placebo, by enhanced suggestion as in hypnosis, or by anxiety reduction as in autohypnosis and natural childbirth training, or it may act as a counter-irritant, or set off the production of endorphins. It is effective in some patients only, varying with their attitude and rapport with acupuncturist and uncertain organic factors.

Behaviour therapy in groups or individually is an integral part of the treatment offered in pain clinics. The aim is to reinforce increased activity and 'well behaviour', and not to reward 'pain behaviour' such as complaints and indications of pain, withdrawal from work and social intercourse (Waddell *et al.*, 1984).

Psychotherapy of the psychoanalytic type helps a minority of patients to understand why they suffer pain and to find other ways of dealing with their neurotic needs.

Transcutaneous nerve stimulation (TNS) is a method of reducing pain input from the periphery, based on the gate theory. Again, it suits some patients.

Biofeedback in which the patient receives information about, for instance, the degree of tension in certain muscles, teaches him to relax them. This manoeuvre is most helpful where muscular tension is producing or enhancing pain, as in neck pain, backache and migraine (see Chapter 16).

REFERENCES

Bond, M.R. (1979) *Pain: its Nature, Analysis and Treatment*, Churchill Livingstone, London

Bradley, L.A. (1983) 'Coping with Chronic Pain', in Burish, T.G. and Bradley, L.A. (Eds) *Coping with Chronic Disease*, Academic Press, New York

Cannon, J.T., Liebeskind, J.C. and Frenk, H. (1978) 'Neural and Neurochemical Mechanisms of Pain Inhibition', in Sternbach, R.A. (Ed.) *The Psychology of Pain*, Raven Press, New York

Fordyce, W.E. (1978) 'Learning Processes in Pain', in Sternbach, R.A. (Ed.), *The Psychology of Pain*, Raven Press, New York

Gomez, J. and Dally, P. (1977) 'Psychologically-mediated Abdominal Pain',

British Medical Journal, 1, 1451-3

Harwood, A. (Ed.) (1981) *Ethnicity and Medical Care*, Harvard University Press, Cambridge, Mass.

Lopez-Ibor, J.J. (1972) 'Masked Depression', *British Journal of Psychiatry*, *120*, 254-7

Melzack, R. and Wall, P.D. (1965) 'Pain Mechanisms: a New Theory', *Science, 150*, 971-8

Merskey, H. (1973) 'The Management of Patients in Pain', *British Journal of Hospital Medicine, 9*, 574-80

Merskey, H. (1976) 'The Status of Pain', from Hill, O.W. (Ed.) *Modern Trends in Psychosomatic Medicine — 3*, Butterworth, London

Pilowsky, I., Chapman, C.R. and Bonica, J.J. (1976) 'Pain, Depression and Illness Behaviour in a Pain Clinic Population', *Pain, 4*, 183-92

Roy, A. (1982) *Hysteria*, Wiley, Chichester and New York

Sinclair, D. (1973) 'The Anatomy and Physiology of Pain', *British Journal of Hospital Medicine, 9*, 568-71

Sternbach, R.A. (1978) 'Clinical Aspects of Pain', in Sternbach, R.A. (Ed.) *The Psychology of Pain*, Raven Press, New York

Trimble, M.R. (1981) 'Chronic Pain' in *Neuropsychiatry*, Wiley, Chichester, and New York

Tyrer, S.P. (1986) 'Learned Pain Behaviour', *British Medical Journal, 292*, 1-2

Waddell, G., Main, C.J., Morriss, E.W., Di Pada, M. and Gray, I.C.M. (1984) 'Chronic Low Back Pain, Psychological Distress and Illness Behaviour' *Spine, 9*, 209-213

5

Liaison in Neurological Disorders

Close association between psychiatry and neurology is personified by that defector from the latter, Sigmund Freud. In ancient Babylon the prestigious priest-physician dealt with mental disorders and internal medicine, whereas lesser, lay practitioners coped with the obvious, for instance injuries. Hippocrates' practice included psychological disorders which he classified into melancholia, mania, paranoia and epilepsy. Despite its Greek origin, psychiatry was not so termed until 1808 by Johann Reil, and the word 'neurologie' was coined by Thomas Willis (1521-1575). Willis also described the limbic system and the localisation of such functions as memory and imagination. In the last half of the nineteenth century, neurology and psychiatry diverged. Wernicke, Alzheimer and Pick each described anatomical lesions associated with disease, and Charcot, Janet and Freud conceptualised the subconscious and suggested mental mechanisms underlying psychiatric illness.

In the last 20 years there has been a rapprochement between the two disciplines, resulting in such hybrid blossoms as neuropsychiatry, neuropsychopharmacology and neuropsychoendocrinology. Since both are rooted in the same physical substrate, it is not surprising that neurological disorders may present with psychiatric symptoms and vice versa, and, in the chronic neurological diseases especially, psychological features are prominent. Kirk and Saunders (1977), examining 2716 patients in a neurological outpatients' department in north-east England, found 13.2 per cent had a primary psychiatric disorder. Of these only 14 per cent had been referred to a psychiatrist. Eighty-two per cent had neuroses or personality disorder, 17 per cent affective disorder, and 1 per cent were schizophrenic. Multiple symptomatology was found in 50 per cent of the 'psychiatric' patients, with headache topping the list of symptoms. Women, far more often than men, suffered blackouts or facial pain. De Paulo and Folstein (1978) found that among neurological inpatients 50 per cent had emotional disorders and 30 per cent cognitive deficits, and in more than 50 per cent of these the symptoms continued throughout the admission. Lipowski and Kiriakos (1972) reviewed 200 neurological inpatients referred to a liaison service. Only 48 per cent of these patients had a definite neurological diagnosis by the time they were discharged, and 38 per cent had both neurological and psychiatric diagnoses. Psychiatric diagnoses comprised: depression 13.5 per cent, organic brain syndroms 20 per cent, schizophrenia 7 per cent and personality disorder 5.5 per cent.

SYMPTOMS

Presenting symptoms in patients who turn out to have major psychiatric problems include headache; pain in the back, face, limbs, neck and trunk; fits, faints and 'funny turns'; dizziness, unsteadiness; movement disorder (tremors, twitches, weakness); paraesthesiae; visual symptoms; aggression and multiple symptoms.

Hysterical conversion symptoms cover all areas: motor symptoms 25 per cent, with tremor an additional 4 per cent; pain 23 per cent; visual disturbances 10 per cent; fits and dizziness 9 per cent; anaesthesia 7 per cent; amnesia 4 per cent. Multiple sclerosis and hysterical symptoms often co-exist. (Trimble, 1981), and it is salutary to remember Slater's dictum that hysteria is 'not only a delusion, but a snare' (Slater and Glithero, 1965). Of 85 patients given a diagnosis of hysteria at the National Hospital for Nervous Diseases, London, follow-up seven to eleven years later revealed 58 per cent to have organic illness and 13 per cent psychiatric illness; 12 per cent had died. Patients with possible neurological disease need particularly careful assessment by the psychiatrist. Disorders of perception may be problematic and will now be discussed.

Auditory perceptual abnormalities

Unformed sounds, such as whistling, clicks or tinnitus, may be heard. These may result from: local middle ear, labyrinthine or eighth-nerve disorders; lesions of the superior temporal gyrus; drug toxicity, for instance with salicylates, quinine and streptomycin; or schizophrenia.

Formed sounds, such as voices or music, may also be due to: end-organ disease; temporal lobe lesions; acute and, less often, chronic organic brain syndromes; hallucinogen effects and amphetamine psychosis; alcoholic hallucinosis; and the functional psychoses.

Tactile perceptual abnormalities

These may occur in diabetes mellitus, cocaine or amphetamine use, hyperventilation, depression, schizophrenia, or monosymptomatic hypochondriasis. Unpleasant interpretations may be put on the perceptions: formication, the feeling of insects crawling on or under the skin, is characteristic of cocaine toxicity, and depressives often believe that they are infested by parasites. A man with monosymptomatic hypochondriasis was convinced that vile insects sucked his blood, and stains from his scratching were 'proof'. Schizophrenics tend to grosser fantasy: one man believed that a rat was gnawing his foot away. On the other hand a patient whose stroke had affected both motor and sensory areas on the right believed that he could feel a large dog dragging him down on that side.

Olfactory perceptual abnormalities

These are usually experienced as unpleasant, for instance 'the smell of death' in schizophrenic or depressive psychoses. Various odours from burning rubber to dead fish may be perceived in complex partial seizures associated with temporal lobe lesions.

Visual perceptual abnormalities

Visual perceptual abnormalities, including flashes, formed hallucinations, macropsia and micropsia, may occur in temporal lobe or occipital lobe disturbance, delirium tremens and other acute organic brain syndromes, hallucinogen and opiate use, functional psychoses and anxiety. Pseudo-hallucinations are most commonly visual: there is a sense of unreality about them. They occur in bereavement and less often in other stressful circumstances in adolescents and those of hysterical personality.

PATIENT ASSESSMENT

In the assessment of a patient with neurological symptoms, as in all liaison work, the history is of paramount significance. Although the general plan (see Chapter 2) should be followed, there are some areas of special relevance:

(1) *Family history* of epilepsy, other neurological disease, mental handicap, diabetes mellitus, early death, dementia. Antenatal and birth complications. Developmental milestones and later academic achievement.

(2) *Occupational history*: exposure to toxic substances such as lead, mercury, disinfectants, weedkillers, pesticides, fungicides and solvents; or exposure in the third world countries to various infections: cerebral malaria, cysticercosis, schistosomiasis, trypanosomiasis and other meningoencephalitides, according to region. Work where alcohol is a commonplace, such as journalism, bartending or being a barrister poses obvious risks. Recurrent head trauma occurs in boxers, wrestlers, jockeys and footballers: the ill-effects may not emerge for many years.

(3) *Past medical history*: significant items are childhood and adult convulsions, head injury, meningitis, migraine, diabetes mellitus, hypertension, overdosage, carbon monoxide poisoning, alcohol and illegal drug use. Anaesthesia for surgery and other possible causes of hypoxia, and any regular medication should be recorded.

(4) *Pending litigation* involving the hope of compensation or the threat of conviction militates against complete recovery, even in the least manipulative of patients. A history of trouble with the police may suggest poor impulse control, disinhibition or undue aggressivity in some cases.

Although physical aspects have a minor part in most psychiatric assessments, in neurological cases a few points are worth noting.

Facial asymmetry may be due to upper or lower motor neurone disease. In the former, which is associated with a contralateral frontal lobe lesion, only the lower part of the face is affected. Spontaneous 'emotional' facial movements may be spared, with the important exception of right-sided frontal tumour. In temporal lobe lesions there is sometimes slight facial asymmetry, and lower motor neurone causes include Bell's palsy and herpes zoster. Functional causes are less persistent and involve muscular spasm rather than weakness.

Abnormal movements of face and body include: senile orofacial dyskinesia; tardive dyskinesia; Parkinson's disease; Huntington's chorea; rheumatic chorea; physiological and familial tremor; Gilles de la Tourette's syndrome and other tics; damage to the cerebellum or basal ganglia from any cause; drug effects, e.g. neuroleptics, tricyclic antidepressants, lithium, levodopa, methyldopa, anti-cholinergics, cocaine and other stimulants; alcohol (withdrawal states and cerebellar damage); and schizophrenia (manneristic and catatonic disorders, tics).

Aphasia, apraxia and agnosia each reflect dysfunction of the cerebral association cortex and are presumptive evidence of organicity. In primary motor aphasia, speech is sparse, hesitant and telegrammatic, with the 'ifs' and 'buts' omitted and incorrect words used, reflecting damage to Broca's area. Writing is impaired, apart from copying. In nominal aphasia the patient cannot put a name to objects, particularly if they are infrequently mentioned, e.g. the *teeth* of a comb, the *milling* on a coin. Unlike primary motor aphasia, it is more often found in diffuse rather than focal dysfunction, for instance in Alzheimer's disease. Acalculia (difficulty with numbers) is a common accompaniment. In sensory or receptive aphasia, comprehension is impaired so that directions are wrongly followed and speech is also impaired: paraphasia and neologisms are frequent but the flow of words is fluent. Lesions in the posterior part of the superior temporal gyrus are likely.

Apraxia is a disorder of skilled movements in any part of the body. It indicates a left parieto-temporal lesion as a rule, but dressing and constructional apraxias are more often associated with right-sided problems, and difficulty in appreciating visuospatial relationships. Agnosia implies difficulty in recognition of objects. Astereognosis is the failure to identify familiar objects by feel, and depends on opposite-side parietal lobe lesions. Colour and visual object agnosias are associated with left occipital lobe defects. The importance of these localising symptoms is in making a correct diagnosis, and in particular not condemning a patient as demented when he has a focal lesion.

Case 1: Mrs B., aged 78, was admitted to hospital after a stroke which left her mildly hemiplegic and apparently unable to understand or complete the simplest of intellectual tests, and talking non-stop nonsense. She was transferred to a psychogeriatric unit as suffering from arteriosclerotic dementia. Her remarkable artistic talents when she got hold of a pencil alerted the staff and closer neuropsychiatric examination showed her to be impaired only in the auditory association cortex in the dominant hemisphere.

Case 2. Mr H., aged 38, was admitted smelling of alcohol and using neologisms and odd phrases strung together without apparent meaning. He also had curious mannerisms, but settled reasonably well into the ward routine. He turned out to be a chronic schizophrenic patient on unofficial leave from a psychiatric hospital.

Primitive reflexes may appear with the ravages of disease and age on the central nervous system. The grasp reflex sought by stroking the palm outwards is associated with disease of the opposite frontal lobe, as is the sucking reflex set off by touching the lips. The palmo-mental reflex, obtained by stroking the thenar eminence, producing wincing on the same side of the chin, is also a harbinger of intellectual deterioration. The glabellar tap test consists of blinking induced by rhythmic tapping on the bridge of the nose: failure to habituate indicates Parkinson's disease.

The senses of smell and taste usually fall off with ageing, rhinitis and smoking, and this has little significance. Unilateral anosmia may indicate compression of the olfactory bulb by a tumour. Visual field defects are of interest: a central scotoma is commonly a sequel to retrobulbar neuritis, which can be due to multiple sclerosis, pernicious anaemia, methyl alcohol, and some pipe tobacco. Bitemporal hemianopia should arouse suspicion of a pituitary tumour. Concentric diminution of the fields is found in severe papilloedema or syphilitic atrophy. Completely tubular vision is usually hysterical. Examination of the optic fundi reveals papilloedema, from raised intracranial pressure, hypertension, polycythaemia vera or, less often, retrobulbar neuritis. A flat, dead-white disc indicates optic atrophy, and in multiple sclerosis the temporal half is strikingly pale, much more obvious than the slight, normal, temporal pallor. Pupil size is reduced in Horner's syndrome and with opiates, pilocarpine and neostigmine, and increased with sympathetic overactivity, atropine and its analogues, cocaine, clomipramine and third nerve lesions. Argyll-Robertson pupils, characteristic of tabes dorsalis and GPI, are small, irregular and unequal, and react to accommodation but not to light. Impaired ocular movements, double vision, lid-lag and nystagmus all require further investigation. Detailed accounts are given by Lishman (1978), Trimble (1981), Roberts (1984) and Walton (1974).

DIAGNOSTIC AIDS IN NEUROLOGY

Diagnostic aids in neurology are reaching increasingly high levels of sophistication and the liaison psychiatrist needs to be aware of them. They include electroencephalography (EEG), computerised axial tomography (CAT scan), positron-emission transaxial tomography (PETT scan), and magnetic resonance imaging (MRI) of the brain. The first is readily and cheaply obtained.

EEG

Basic characteristics to remember are the frequencies: delta, less than 4 Hz, theta 4-7 Hz, alpha 8-13 Hz, beta, more than 13 Hz. In normal adults with eyes closed the alpha rhythm is predominant, and maximal in parietal and occipital regions. It attenuates with eye opening and mental activity. The average voltage is 30-50 μV, which is reduced with relaxation and drowsiness. Rhythms of less than 4 Hz are pathological, and those of 4-8 Hz may represent either immaturity, ageing or pathology. Fast rhythms are frequently due to drug administration, for instance benzodiazepines. In normal sleep the EEG slows progressively to 1-2 Hz, with superimposed 'spindles' of 14 Hz activity. In rapid eye movement (REM) sleep, the EEG desynchronises and shows eye-movement artefacts. Apart from slow rhythms, the indicators of epilepsy are the most important features to look for in the EEG: generalised or focal spikes or sharp waves, and paroxysms of spike and wave complexes. In *petit mal* epilepsy, 3 Hz and wave discharges are characteristic during an attack, and may be induced, as may other epileptic activity, by hyperventilation and other causes of cerebral hypoxia, or by photic stimulation.

Marked asymmetry of EEG activity between the hemispheres indicates organicity, as does a single focus of slow (or, occasionally, fast) activity. In the hyperventilation syndrome the symptoms are reproduced during overbreathing, but the EEG shows no epileptic discharge. Despite its limitations, since 12-15 per cent of normal adults have abnormal traces, and there are variations with level of arousal, blood glucose and acid-base equilibrium, the EEG is useful.

Uses of the EEG in neuropsychiatry

The EEG can be used for diagnosis in epilepsy; hyperventilation syndrome; acute organic brain syndromes, especially hepatic coma; dementia, especially Huntington's chorea or rapidly progressive disease; rapidly progressing tumour; and drugs, especially barbiturates.

The EEG helps in excluding organicity in depression, fits, post-traumatic syndrome, stupor and catatonia.

Medication affects the EEG variously. Benzodiazepines,

barbiturates, phenothiazines, primidone and most antidepressants except viloxazine enhance epileptic activity. Fast activity appears with most sedatives, and slow waves are produced by high doses of phenothiazines and tricyclic antidepressants. Electroconvulsive therapy leads to slow waves with frontal preponderance becoming more marked with further treatments, and persisting for up to two months.

Functional psychiatric disorders provide disappointingly non-specific EEG abnormalities. Those with personality disorders, particularly aggressive sociopaths, have immature EEGs in 60 per cent, involving the posterior part of the temporal lobes in particular. Some schizophrenics also show temporal lobe abnormalities, but of the epileptic type, and paroxysms of fast or slow activity.

CAT Scans

CAT scans of the head show up structural alterations and disorders of the normal brain architecture. Ventricular enlargement and cortical atrophy occur in progressive organic brain syndromes such as Alzheimer's disease or in diabetes mellitus or chronic alcoholism. Displacement of normal structures may be due to space-occupying lesions or contracting scar tissue. Tumours, demyelination and blood vessel abnormalities may require contrast enhancement to be seen. In time, apparent atrophy in alcoholics and patients with Cushing's disease or severe anorexia nervosa may recover.

PETT brain scans

PETT brain scans give information on regional cerebral blood flow (rCBF) and metabolism. Advance warning of Huntington's chorea can be obtained without alarming the patient as in the levodopa challenge test; schizophrenics tend to a reduction in frontal blood flow (Buchsbaum et al., 1982).

MRI

MRI of the brain is particularly useful in differentiating white and gray matter, and promises to be useful in the diagnosis of demyelinating disease.

NEUROLOGICAL DISORDERS WITH PROMINENT PSYCHOLOGICAL COMPONENTS

These include: epilepsy, Huntington's chorea, multiple sclerosis, Parkinson's disease, cerebral syphilis, trigeminal neuralgia and other facial pain, cerebrovascular disease, brain tumour and other masses, alcohol-related neurological disorders, Wernicke's encephalopathy, subarachnoid haemorrhage, motor neurone disease, migraine and other headaches, and post-traumatic syndromes.

EPILEPSY

Epilepsy is to neurology what schizophrenia is to psychiatry: an important, relatively common, chronic disorder, varying in type and symptomatology, disruptive to the patient's life — and difficult to define. It is characterised by fits: sudden, episodic disturbances of function in the central nervous system, prone to recur. The essence of a fit or seizure is an abnormal and excessive discharge of neurones in the brain, which may be few and localised or many and widespread.

There are various types of seizure: simple partial fits (with no loss of consciousness), which are motor, sensory, autonomic, and rarely psychic; and complex partial fits (with impaired consciousness), usually involving one or both temporal lobes. Partial seizures may progress to generalised, i.e. absences (interrupted consciousness), with or without motor or autonomic components — *petit mal*; or tonic-clonic fits (loss of consciousness), i.e. *grand mal*.

Grand mal

The classic fit begins suddenly: the patient falls, perhaps with a single cry, and, after a transient stage of maximal tonus, there follows a minute or two of interrupted, fading tonus (the clonic stage). The patient is unconscious, his pupils are dilated, his plantar reflexes are extensor; he remains unrousable for from a few minutes to as long as an hour, then passes through a stage of confusion. This has the hallmarks of an acute organic brain syndrome and may pass within a few minutes or continue for a week or more. By this time the neurologists will have asked for a psychiatric opinion.

71

Obviously the postictal course depends upon the cause of the fit, and the state of the patient's brain. Recovery is slow in the elderly, alcoholic and otherwise brain-impaired, and occasionally progresses directly from an acute to a chronic brain syndrome: for instance in a presenile dementia.

The causes of epilepsy to consider include direct genetic loading or the indirect influence of such heredofamilial disorders as phenylketonuria, epiloia, and antenatal or birth complications. Causes acquired later are: head trauma, which particularly affects the temporal lobes; alcohol, lead and other toxicity; drug effects with, for instance, phenothiazines or tricyclic antidepressants and withdrawal from sedatives such as alcohol, barbiturates and lorazepam; metabolic and endocrine upsets, including uraemia and hypoglycaemia; and structural changes from cerebrovascular disease, tumour and degenerative disorders, especially Alzheimer's disease.

The precipitants of a seizure in the susceptible may be emotional stress, lack of sleep, fever, hypoxia from any cause, and hyperventilation. Reflex epilepsies may be recognised by their regular occurrence after the specific stimulus, which might be anything from light on water, music, or mental arithmetic to orgasm.

The psychiatrist is often consulted when there is a doubt whether a patient's attacks are genuine epileptic fits. Other organic causes of falling to the ground should be borne in mind: myasthenia gravis, transient vertebrobasilar ischaemia, familial periodic paralysis, cataplexy in narcoleptics, and normal pressure hydrocephalus: none of these involves loss of consciousness. Falls with unconsciousness may be faints due to temporary failure of the cerebral circulation, as in heart-block or other cardiovascular problems; micturition or cough syncope in the over 50s; the first half of pregnancy; anaemia; pain or emotional shock; and rarely, in adolescence, focal vertebrobasilar migraine.

Hysterical fits

Like other conversion phenomena, these serve two purposes: immediate escape from stress or anxiety, and secondary rewards. They may be suspected if the patient reiterates how much he or she wants to get on with his life, emphasising simultaneously that his severe incapacity makes it quite impossible. To complicate the issue it is not uncommon for hysterical fits to occur in patients who have *grand mal* seizures also. Such patients are often those of limited intellectual gifts and interrupted education who are having problems with employment and in their personal relations (Roy, 1977). The characteristics of *grand mal* and hysterical fits are compared in Table 5.1.

Table 5.1: Characteristics of *Grand Mal* and Hysterical Fits

One cry at onset, if at all	May moan or scream
Stereotyped tonic-clonic sequence	Often thrashing about
Loss of consciousness	Variable: may be able to remember events during fit
May bite tongue severely	Rarely bites tongue
May be incontinent	Rarely incontinent
Extensor plantars	Normal plantars
Characteristic EEG changes during fit	EEG may be abnormal
Serum prolactin level raised after fit	Not raised, unless patient on phenothiazines or tricyclics
Fit may occur in sleep	Never in sleep
May be pale or cyanosed	Pallor common
Confusion follows fit	May have no confusion
Seldom more than once in 24 hours	May occur several times daily

If a patient is considered to be having hysterical fits, it must be remembered that these are unconsciously mediated and he requires compassionate handling. Apart from their intrinsic primary anxiety, such patients are often depressed and have emotional and social problems which need attention. Malingering is rare.

Complex partial seizures

Fits originating in temporal lobe foci or those in the adjoining frontal and occipital lobes exciting the temporal area secondarily may manifest in seemingly psychiatric symptoms. Some of the abnormalities of perception have been reviewed: epileptic hallucinations, with the exception of those of smell, are oddly devoid of affect. Brief, episodic abnormalities of thought, mood, behaviour and consciousness also occur, for instance 'forced thinking', in which an unbidden thought dominates the mind; inexplicable panic, depression or euphoria; and lip-smacking, chewing, running or laughing. Dysphasia is present in 20 per cent of temporal lobe epileptics, and their search for the right words may account in part for their circumstantiality.

Automatisms are quasi-purposeful actions, rarely violent, intrinsic to or following a fit, and are carried out in a state of altered consciousness. They rarely last more than 15 minutes, but it is possible for complex partial seizures to continue as a form of status epilepticus. Violence associated with epilepsy is usually random and unpremeditated, and the patient takes no precautions to guard himself against injury or being caught. He can seldom remember the episode. If violent crime is committed by a sufferer from epilepsy, it is unlikely to result from his disease.

Psychosocial concomitants of epilepsy

Fits are embarrassing to contemplate, and involve a risk of injury as well as a restriction in work, sport and travel. The prejudice against epileptics is worse than that against psychiatric patients (Bagley, 1972): friendships and sexual relationships may be difficult. This may be enhanced by the attitude of passive dependence inculcated by protective parents and institutions, and for women by the knowledge that their babies run an increased risk of cleft lip and palate. Intellectual impairment, slow learning and poor memory may result from the underlying brain lesion and additionally the effect of chronic medication. The epileptic is likely to find himself less well educated, and in a poorly paid, unstimulating and isolated job.

Petit mal in children interferes with their learning, so they do badly in school. They have been shown by Stores (1978) to be unduly distractible, overactive, deviant, socially isolated and dependent on their mothers. Prejudicial factors are male sex, a father doing manual work, and a left temporal lobe lesion.

Neurotic disorders

Conduct disorders were noted by Rutter *et al.* (1970) to be four times more likely to occur in epileptic children than in others. In adult patients persistent mild depression or anxiety occur in one-third, with hysterical conversion symptoms in a proportion of these. Explanation, social support and individual or mixed-sex, mixed-diagnosis group psychotherapy are useful in these patients.

Sexual problems

Contralateral genital sensations may occur as seizure phenomena in medial temporal lesions, and temporal lobectomy is reported to be associated with cases of fetishism and transvestism (Scott, 1978). However, the common complaints of low libido and impotence are partly due to low self-esteem, and also can be an indirect effect of anticonvulsant therapy. Enhanced liver enzymes metabolise testosterone unduly quickly (Toone *et al.*, 1980).

Personality problems

The stereotype of the epileptic personality characterised by pedantry, religiosity, circumstantiality, egocentricity and suspiciousness would equally well fit many chronic schizophrenics, institutionalised by their illness in a hospital, a hostel or at home. Lishman (1978) and Scott (1978) consider that there is no specific personality disorder associated with epilepsy. Nevertheless, at the Maudsley Hospital (London), among other specialist clinics, 60 per cent of epileptic admissions are considered to have a primary personality disorder, mainly of the passive dependent type. Bear and Fedio (1977) hypothesise an enhanced affective association with otherwise neutral stimuli in temporal lobe epilepsy, so that patients may explain commonplace events and activities in religious or mystical terms in their striving after meaning. The authors suggest that patients with left-sided foci are particularly prone to these traits, and to hypergraphia, whereas those with right temporal lobe involvement are more overtly emotional. Explosive aggressiveness has been considered a feature of the epileptic personality but there are no methodologically sound studies, and many deprivation factors are involved (Fenton, 1983).

Psychoses

A clouded state may occur in *petit mal* status, resembling presenile dementia in those of middle age. Continuous spike and wave patterning in the EEG nails the diagnosis. Psychomotor complex partial status by contrast is extremely rare. Postictal confusional states are classic acute organic brain syndromes (see Chapter 3) and may follow any type of seizure. They are commoner in males and when there is a fit frequency of more than one a week. The clouding results from diffuse inhibition of neuronal function, reflected in slowing of the EEG rhythms; it may last minutes, hours, even weeks.

Interictal psychoses

These are not time-related to individual seizures and arise in clear consciousness. They present either as a major affective illness, usually depressive, or a schizophrenia-like state of paranoid style. As Flor-Henry (1969) and more recently Perez *et al.* (1985) have argued, the laterality of the temporal lobe focus probably determines the symptom complex: schizophrenia-like with dominant, affective with non-dominant hemisphere involvement. Importantly, from the point of view of treatment, they do not have the transience of fit-related phenomena. It appears that von Meduna's (1937) observation that paranoid psychotic symptoms often subside with increased fit frequency and vice versa has been misinterpreted as an antagonism between schizophrenia and epilepsy. Wolf and Trimble (1985) have reviewed the evidence. The paranoid psychoses of epilepsy are chronic, and in Beard and Slater's study (1962) the cardinal symptoms of schizophrenia were manifest. The differences between these patients and a non-epileptic schizophrenic population included absence of premorbid schizoid traits, maintenance of affective responsivity and rapport, negative psychiatric family history and a strong predominance of paranoid presentations, often with a religious flavor. Onset was insidious, and the mean period since the start of the epilepsy was 14 years. Treatment with neuroleptics is successful in these cases, but the potential epileptogenicity of such drugs may lead to an increase in fit frequency and the anticonvulsant dosage needs increasing. However, if phenytoin is used, phenothiazines and tricyclics increase its plasma level, occasionally leading to intoxication.

Depression is the commonest psychiatric illness associated with epilepsy, particularly temporal lobe epilepsy, but this is usually neurotic. Whitlock (1982) suggests that 15-40 per cent of temporal lobe epileptics suffer from severe affective psychoses, some of manic-depressive symptomatology and periodicity, others of the schizo-affective type. Treatment with antidepressant or neuroleptic medication must be given, checking anticonvulsant needs. Nomifensine, which raises the epileptic threshold, has been suggested as suitable in depressed epileptics, but this has now been withdrawn (Gomez, 1985).

Suicide is an appreciable risk in epileptics: Whitlock (1977) found that 6.5 per cent of suicides in England and Wales occurred in patients with neurological disease, and of these 27 per cent were epileptic. Attempted suicide is also particularly common in epileptics (Hawton et al., 1980); some are no doubt due to impulsive acts, but others are the result of serious affective disorder.

'Epileptic dementia', i.e. chronic and progressive deterioration of intellectual, personality and social capability, occurs in a minority of patients. It may be the end-state in a schizophrenia-like psychosis, or result from repeated anoxia or an underlying brain lesion. Pond (1957) found a group suffering from neurotic withdrawal but presenting with pseudo-dementia. CAT scanning is indicated if in doubt.

HUNTINGTON'S CHOREA

This dreadful disease encompassing madness, bizarre movements, dementia and early death affects the sexes equally, with a worldwide prevalence of 4-7 per 100 000. An abnormal gene on the short arm of chromosome 4 is transmitted as an autosomal dominant of high penetrance so that 50 per cent of the children of a patient will develop the disease (Harper, 1983). It commonly presents in the fourth decade, but in 10-20 per cent onset is in childhood, and occasionally past 50. The movement disorder may be misinterpreted in the early stages as fidgetiness or tics, and patients are adept at incorporating involuntary movements into purposeful acts. A minority develop muscular weakness before any noticeable movement disorder (Caine and Shoulson, 1983).

Half the patients first come to notice because of psychiatric abnormalities. *Personality problems* may be the first indication: disinhibition leads to coarseness, promiscuity or aggression, and an awkward 'don't care' attitude in work and at home. Alcohol or cannabis misuse may crop up (Dewhurst, 1970).

> *Case*: Mr M. is in frequent trouble with the police for public sexual approaches to men, women and children and on one occasion dented a middle-aged lady's car when she refused him a lift.

A schizophrenia-like psychosis seems a natural progression in some cases. The prime symptoms are grandiose and persecutory delusions, and in 15 per cent auditory hallucinations.

Depression of the reactive type is understandable in Huntington's chorea, but in 17 per cent of patients a psychotic depression arises, also with persecutory delusions. Suicide is a substantial risk (Trimble, 1981; Koehler and Sass, 1984).

Dementia sets in in 66 per cent of Huntington's chorea patients. It has a characteristic pattern, starting with memory difficulties, loss of insight and judgement, and poor concentration. Disorientation and dysphasia are not features, and the picture resembles the frontal lobe syndrome of impaired cortical executive function. Death usually comes within 15 years of the onset of the disease, and a family history of early death is significant.

The liaison psychiatrist may be asked to help with the diagnosis if the typical combination of choreiform movements, psychiatric disorder and family history is absent. Tests for a genetic marker are not yet established, EEG abnormalities of low voltage alpha rhythm may not show, and the levodopa challenge may alarm by inducing involuntary movements. CAT scanning may provide useful evidence of shrinkage of the caudate nuclei and often cortical atrophy, and a PETT scan shows reduced blood flow in this area very early.

Treatment of the unwanted movements — and to some extent unacceptable impulses — is achieved with tetrabenazine (up to 200 mg daily in divided doses: not available in the US) and/or haloperidol (10-80 mg daily in divided doses) which induce extrapyramidal rigidity. They are also depressant. The psychiatric manifestations are treated symptomatically with medication or electroconvulsive therapy. Special hostel or other institutional care is likely to be necessary ultimately. An onerous duty is counselling the patient and his relatives on the genetic disorder; voluntary support associations offer help to those who will accept it (Saugstad and Odegard, 1986).

MULTIPLE SCLEROSIS

This strange, demoralising disease commonly presents in the third or fourth decade with an odd mix of apparently unconnected neurological symptoms. These are usually short-lived and may be triggered by such somatic stress as acute infection, inoculation or pregnancy. The course of the illness is irregularly fluctuant, with symptomatic remissions lasting perhaps for years, during a downhill progression. Some 15 per cent do not remit (Trimble, 1981). The cause of the disease is unclear, but the pathology has been established of patchy demyelination and plaque formation anywhere in the spinal cord, brainstem, cranial nerves, cerebellum and cerebral hemispheres. Charcot's triad of cerebellar effects is sometimes seen: nystagmus, tremor and scanning speech. Other symptoms include diplopia, blurred vision, vertigo, weakness, spasticity, pain or paraesthesiae, impotence and bladder dysfunction, at any time, in any order. Such manifestations, particularly as they seem impermanent, may be misread as hysterical and indeed, as with epilepsy, patients with multiple sclerosis not uncommonly present both hysterical and organically mediated symptoms.

Psychological aspects of the disease

These may be affective or organic. Twenty-five per cent show depression with anxiety, usually of the reactive type. This may precede the neurological presentation in 7 per cent of cases. There is an increased risk of suicide (Kahana *et al.*, 1971). Euphoria has been described as characteristic of multiple sclerosis (Surridge, 1969). Rarely it may indicate the hysterical defence of denial of illness, but usually it is due to a dementing process affecting in particular the frontal lobes, or it is possibly a response to corticosteroids, frequently administered in the acute phases of the illness. Progressive organic deterioration of intellectual and personality functions is not usually obvious until 50 ml of brain substance is out of service. Memory impairment and emotional lability are likely in multiple sclerosis. A severe pathological exaggeration and prolongation of laughing and crying occurs if the corticobulbar tracts are affected on both sides. Pseudobulbar palsy, producing spastic dysarthria and dysphagia, may arise in multiple sclerosis and multi-infarct dementia, but not in Alzheimer's or Parkinson's disease (Folstein and McHugh, 1983).

The liaison psychiatrist's chief concerns are diagnosis, absolute and proportional — the input of organic and psychological factors, respectively — and management. Clinical examination includes the psychiatric and neurological, with special reference to the dead-white temporal pallor indicative of previous optic neuritis seen in 70 per cent of cases of multiple sclerosis. Visual evoked potentials also reveal optic neuritis in delayed responses and asymmetry, and the test is positive in up to 90 per cent of cases. Lumbar puncture shows a cluster of abnormalities in the cerebrospinal fluid, none specific, and the electroencephalogram may show focal or diffuse slowing.

Treatment

Neurological treatments include linoleic acid, immunosuppression, and, in the acute stage, ACTH. Diazepam (20-40 mg daily in divided doses) baclofen (20-80 mg daily in divided doses) and physiotherapy are useful when there is spasticity, but both the muscle relaxants are mildly depressant. The psychiatrist should be prepared to offer or arrange supportive psychotherapy for depression, anxiety and sexual problems, and relatives may also need counselling. Medication may help to alleviate depression and anxiety, for instance dothiepin (50-150 mg divided or at night), maprotiline (50-150 mg divided or at night). Dothiepin is not available in the US, but imipramine in the same dosage may be substituted or tranylcypromine (10-40 mg daily, before 4 pm): both drugs are non-sedating. For problematic disinhibition, haloperidol (3-40 mg daily, divided) is useful, or thioridazine (25-100 mg daily, in divided doses) in organically produced agitation.

PARKINSONISM

Parkinsonism may be a primary disorder or secondary to medication, especially neuroleptics, cerebrovascular disease or encephalitis lethargica. In 1817 James Parkinson described the disorder as characterised by tremor, weakness and a festinant gait, but wrongly believed the intellect to be unscathed. Idiopathic parkinsonism usually presents between 50 and 59 years, and is likely to be more rapidly progressive if it manifests before 40. Men are affected slightly more often than women and there is a hereditary tendency. Most patients have to stop work four years after onset, but life expectancy has increased from ten to fourteen years since the introduction of levodopa.

The underlying pathology involves neuronal deterioration and loss in the substantia nigra, and, significantly, neurofibrillary tangles, senile plaques and granulovacuolar degeneration as in Alzheimer's disease.

Subtle psychiatric and obvious neurological symptoms usually come on simultaneously, hence the traditional antidepressant/anticholinergic cocktail. Up to 60 per cent of patients present as clinically depressed, and in 17 per cent there is tremor at rest of the hands ('pill-rolling') or jaw at a frequency of 4-8 cycles per second. It may be unilateral initially. Rigidity, with 'lead-pipe' or 'cogwheel' quality on examination, affects both agonist and antagonist groups of muscles, and unlike the tremor this persists during sleep. Poverty and slowness of movement produce a mask-like face with little blinking, crabbed writing, difficulty in initiating any movement, and a shuffling gait. Hypokinesia may be abolished temporarily by fear or excitement. The trunk is bent forwards, displacing the centre of gravity and inducing a tendency to run and to fall. Difficulty in swallowing may lead to excess saliva in the mouth. Constipation is a major nuisance, seborrhoea a minor one.

Secondary parkinsonism

Drug-induced parkinsonism usually arises within two months of starting neuroleptic medication, and tends to subside over time on the same dosage. In some patients parkinsonian symptoms linger on for weeks or months after the drug is stopped. Rigidity is more apparent than tremor in drug-induced cases. In post-encephalitic parkinsonism there is a particular proneness to oculogyric crises and the prognosis is good, whereas in the variety associated with cerebrovascular disease the outlook is poor.

Treatment

In the past 15 years, treatment in Parkinson's disease has undergone a revolution. Anticholinergic drugs, such as benzhexol, benztropine and procyclidine, are still useful in early cases, but a giant leap in progress has been the introduction of levodopa, usually given with a decarboxylase inhibitor to reduce gastric irritation. It replaces a physiological deficiency of dopamine. Seventy per cent of patients show improvement within the first month, but in two years only 60 per cent still benefit, and in six years 50 per cent have given up the medication because of the side-effects. These are usually psychiatric. Amantidine, which loses its efficacy over a few weeks, and bromocriptine are alternatives. The least damaging neuroleptics, if these are necessary, are thioridazine (30-200 mg daily) and sulpiride (400-800 mg daily): use the minimum effective dosage. Sulpiride is not yet freely available in the US.

Psychiatric aspects

Depression is occasionally diagnosed before the neurological symptoms are overt, but usually accompanies them. Tricyclic antidepressants, such as imipramine (75-150 mg daily), are moderately effective.

Cognitive deterioration is not surprising in view of the histopathology, and after six years of levodopa one-third of patients are obviously demented (*British Medical Journal*, 1981). This may be due to their increased age — enhanced life-expectancy correlates with continued taking of levodopa — or perhaps the drug tends to flog the brain to exhaustion, as tolbutamide does to the pancreas. The on-off phenomenon in which the patient alternates willy-nilly between activity and immobility may be an indication of this. Slowness and apathy but not aphasia characterise parkinsonian intellectual fall-off, and there is often cortical atrophy and ventricular enlargement in these cases. Because of the risk that levodopa may increase the likelihood of dementia, it is wise to delay starting it until the patient's discomfort demands its use.

Confusional states with hallucinations, nightmares, excitement and sometimes paranoid ideation may be induced by any of the drugs in use for parkinsonism: anticholinergics, levodopa, amantidine and bromocriptine. Manic states occur occasionally.

Visual hallucinations, often of strange people such as dwarfs or leprechauns, may occur in the daytime or at night regardless of treatment. There is usually an element of insight, and the patient would like to be rid of them. Unfortunately neither neuroleptics nor other psychotropic medication helps. Psychotherapeutic and social support for patients and relatives is likely to be necessary in the later stages of the illness (Ridley *et al.*, 1986).

CEREBRAL SYPHILIS

Although syphilis is far less prevalent than 50 years ago, the incidence has remained steady since 1960 at 20 000 new cases annually in the United States (Tramont, 1979). Neurosyphilis is a late result of the infection and it is important to bear this in mind since its effects are so devastating without treatment. By the time the symptoms of neurosyphilis emerge, the original infection has been forgotten — if the patient was ever aware of it. Thirty-three per cent of Tramont's new cases were in homosexuals, especially in non-white groups, and in anal intercourse a passive partner may not realise that he has acquired an infection. If he has been living in a country where antibiotics are less readily available than in the West, he may not have had a course for a sore throat or other infection, which might incidentally have dealt with his syphilis. The most likely victim of cerebral syphilis today is a homosexual man in his thirties or forties, who has spent some time in the third world.

Subacute and chronic meningovascular syphilis

This arises one to five years after the primary episode, as a secondary or tertiary manifestation. Pathologically it comprises diffuse inflammatory thickening of the meninges with areas of necrosis. The onset of symptoms may be deceptively insidious and intermittent, with localised headaches, lethargy and malaise. The patient becomes slow, forgetful and irritable; his concentration and judgement decline, giving way to increasing emotionality, episodes of clouding and even frank delirium. Cranial nerve disturbances appear. Serological tests are positive in the blood but the cerebrospinal fluid may show only a moderate increase in cells.

Tabes dorsalis

This is associated with general paresis in 20 per cent of cases, and is important in alerting the physician to the likelihood of the latter. It arises 8-12 years after infection, most often in males. The basic lesion is atrophy of the dorsal roots and posterior columns of the spinal cord. The symptoms are startling but creep up gradually: 'lightning pains' and paraesthesiae in the legs; sensory ataxia with a high-stepping gait; and 'crises' of visceral pain. These may last several days and involve the stomach, bladder or larynx. The limb joints may become disorganised.

Psychiatric symptoms develop late: commonly a paranoid or depressive psychosis. Sensory and pupillary abnormalities are present in 90 per cent of cases of tabes, and tests of blood and cerebrospinal fluid confirm the diagnosis.

General paresis (GPI)

This quaternary manifestation of syphilis appears 10-15 years after the primary stage. *Treponema pallidum* can be demonstrated in the brain, which is shrunken especially in the frontal and parietal regions, and encased in thickened meninges. Presenting features more often seem psychiatric than neurological, and may reflect frontal lobe involvement. Alterations in personality, moodiness and outbursts of temper may be noticed by others, and the patient may complain of headaches, insomnia and sometimes unaccustomed difficulty with numbers. More often a sudden episode of memory loss sounds the first warning.

Case: A salesman, aged 38, forgot where he had left the firm's car, and the following week could not remember his own address.

Judgement may unexpectedly fail, as in a man who ordered 700 hymn books for 16 people (Lishman, 1978).

Depression is the commonest presentation currently, at 27 per cent. The patient is slow and silent, and may have nihilistic delusions. In Dewhurst's sample of 91 patients, five presented with a suicidal attempt (Dewhurst, 1969). ECT must never be given in this situation of active brain infection. Even in depression, affect may seem curiously shallow because of the developing dementia. The Victorian-style onset of GPI, with grandiose delusions (Beccle, 1946), is now rare and if it arises is more in keeping with a frontal lobe syndrome, with a quality of naivety. Insight is lost early in the dementing process, with reduction of interests and retardation. Quiet, unnoticed deterioration is frequently brought to light by a startling social lapse.

A common neurological onset is with a *grand mal* seizure, and neurological features in a developed case include: pupillary abnormalities, sometimes of the Argyll-Robertson type; coarse, irregular tremor of face, tongue and hands; and dysarthria. Laboratory tests underpin the diagnosis.

Treatment

At worst, treatment will halt the destructive processes of neurosyphilis, and may lead to a degree of recovery especially in meningovascular disease. It should normally be supervised by a specialist in genitourinary medicine, along such guidelines as those of the US Public Health Service. Parenteral penicillin is usually given, with care for the Herxheimer reaction of pyrexia and enhanced symptoms. Tetracycline or erythromycin may be used in the penicillin sensitive. Psychotropic medication has no special place except for difficult organic symptoms requiring neuroleptics, but some patients with an irrecoverable chronic brain syndrome may require long-term psychiatric hospitalisation.

FACIAL PAIN

Diagnoses which have usually been excluded before a liaison request for persistent facial pain is made are local infection, temporomandibular arthritis, parotid disease, cranial arteritis and post-herpetic neuralgia. Migrainous neuralgia (cluster headache) commonly affects young men. Unilateral pain in eye, cheek and temple, with running nose and eye on the same side, recurs at 24-hour intervals, each attack lasting an hour or two. Ergotamine provides dramatic relief.

Trigeminal neuralgia (tic douloureux) and atypical facial pain both tend to affect the over-fifties. The former consists of 20-second paroxysms of acute pain, 'like red-hot bullets', triggered by external stimuli in the Vth nerve area, e.g.contact,a cold wind, or movement as in yawning. Male patients will not shave during an attack, and female patients will not make-up; both protect the face without touching it. Carbamazepine usually brings relief, but surgical intervention may be necessary. A typical facial pain, by contrast usually occurs in women, often the bereaved, and comprises continuous aching in face, teeth and sometimes neck and arm during the waking hours. Even if the patient denies depression, she is likely to suffer disturbed sleep and feel 'dreadful' in the mornings. She is usually well groomed and not afraid to touch the painful parts. Analgesics are ineffective in this predominantly affective disorder, but antidepressants, either tricyclics or MAOIs, may be most helpful and open the way to discussion of the patient's loneliness or other fears.

CEREBROVASCULAR DISORDERS

When emboli, thromboses or haemorrhage affect the brain in a focal fashion, a range of deficits may occur, alone or in combination, similarly to the situation in multiple sclerosis: for instance dysphasia, dysarthria, dyspraxia, cortical blindness, and amnesia or frontal syndromes. Multi-infarct dementia is often ushered in by transient episodes of weakness or sensory loss. It is likely to develop in a setting of hypertension or atherosclerosis, and is characterised by stepwise patchy deterioration. Insight is often preserved, with resultant reactive depression.

Major cerebrovascular accidents may lead to an immediate acute organic brain syndrome with disorientation, delusional ideas and abnormal affect (Cutting,1983). After this subsides leaving more or less obvious organic impairment, for example in speech and movement, other psychiatric sequelae may emerge. Personality changes following stroke include irritability and aggression: a well-brought-up lady may hit out at the smallest provocation. Equally distressing to relatives and professionals are apathy and withdrawal. Clinical depression is frequent, particularly in patients with right-sided lesions, with tense, perfectionist premorbid personalities, and suffering from severe frustration just before the stroke. The common organic lability of emotional expression, with easy weeping, should not be misinterpreted as depression. Folstein *et al.* (1977) advocate antidepressant treatment in post-stroke depression, but tricyclics in particular, if given too soon, may act as cerebral irritants and increase the tendency to confusion or precipitate a fit.

Barriers to rehabilitation with which the psychiatrist may be able to help with medication and supportive or behavioural psychotherapy include depressive disorders with negativism, lack of confidence and short attention span. Some patients who are suspected of 'not trying' have right-sided lesions with visuospatial defects, disturbed body image or difficulties in comprehension.

Subarachnoid haemorrhage

This accounts for 8 per cent of cerebrovascular catastrophes and unlike other strokes affects those of any age including childhood, but most commonly between 40 and 60. Sixty per cent result from ruptured intracranial aneurysm; in others there is no structural lesion. Rarely the cause is a hypertensive crisis in a patient on an MAOI who has taken cheese or a sympathomime. Onset of subarachnoid haemorrhage is abrupt with intense occipital pain. Some patients rapidly lose consciousness, but others — of interest to the psychiatrist — behave in a bizarre fashion and may be diagnosed as drunk, on drugs or hysterical. Extensor plantar reflexes and severe neck stiffness are the alarm signals for urgent neurological/neurosurgical care. Storey (1972) in his six-year follow-up study found increased irritability, anxiety and apathy to be common complaints. Those with anterior cerebral or communicating artery aneurysms were sometimes reported as improved in personality: less tense and irritable. Some became disinhibited.

BRAIN TUMOURS AND OTHER MASSES

Despite the neurotic fear of some patients with tension headaches, the chances are about 500 to one against headache being the primary presentation of brain tumour. *Slow-growing* tumours lead to personality changes in the direction of the patient's permorbid propensities, with impaired responsiveness and sometimes peevishness. *Moderately progressive* tumours are associated with cognitive deficits, for instance in memory and judgement, and general slowing. *Rapidly growing* tumours cause acute organic reactions, such as seizures, with obvious impairment of consciousness.

In general, psychiatric symptoms are more likely with a glioma than a meningioma, with a glioblastoma than an astrocytoma, and with malignant rather than benign growths. Multiple, small, bilateral metastases are particularly prone to produce mental manifestations.

The characteristics of brain tumours vary enormously with individual patterns of response, often merely exaggerating a trait already present. Fluctuations in the dynamics of the cerebrospinal fluid circulation disturb the level of consciousness. Subtle early changes are occasional lapses of memory or of concentration and rather ready mental fatigue. Somnolence comes on at a later stage, leading finally into coma. Focal cognitive changes may appear even when consciousness is unimpaired, for instance dysphasias or dyspraxias; or there may be a mild dementia with concrete thinking, slowness and improverishment. Affective changes range from depression to euphoria, obsessionality to apathy. Fleeting delusions, organic excitement, and hallucinations in any modality may all arise with brain tumour.

Frontal tumours are notorious deceivers of both psychiatrists and neurologists and there is a plethora of documented cases of patients incarcerated for many years in a mental hospital with a frontal meningioma. Early symptoms are a varying degree of disinhibition, leading to socially unacceptable manners: fatuousness, facetiousness, familiarity, and finally apathy. Urinary and faecal incontinence develop early, and ataxic gait comes later. Temporal lobe tumours often involve intellectual fall-off, especially if they are on the left, and a frontal lobe personality. Fifty per cent of patients have fits, and a few have schizophrenia-like symptoms with auditory or visual hallucinations. Pathognomonic of a temporal lobe lesion are visual hallucinations in a hemianopic field of vision. Parietal lobe tumours have interesting localising neurological symptoms, such as disturbances of body image and neglect of one side with right-sided lesions, and with dominant lesions dysphasia and components of the Gerstmann syndrome. These are finger agnosia, dyscalculia, dyspraxia and right-left disorientation. Mental symptoms are seldom seen in occipital tumours, although difficulties in visual recognition may not be recognised as organic.

Diencephalic tumours, particularly if they involve structures near the 3rd ventricle, may be misinterpreted. An amnestic syndrome with confabulation can occur without the usual alcohol excess of Korsakov's psychosis. Thermoregulation may be upset, eating and drinking patterns may be grossly disturbed, narcolepsy may come on, and impotence and amenorrhoea are common.

Case: A newly married young woman was considered to be showing a hysterical reaction when she began eating and drinking insatiably and turned the fires full on in a heat wave. She had a glioma infiltrating the wall of the 3rd venticle.

Pituitary tumours may present with raised intracranial pressure, visual failure or symptoms of pituitary dysfunction which in turn causes psychiatric symptoms: see Chapter 9.

In brain tumour, abscess or chronic subdural haematoma, the psychiatrist's first task is to assist in diagnosis using the methods mentioned earlier and, as an initial screen, skull X-ray. Displacement of the pineal gland, calcification in a tumour, or localised bone change demands further study. Symptomatic psychotropic medication may be needed, and if the patient is aware of his plight, psychotherapeutic support.

ALCOHOL-RELATED NEUROLOGICAL DISORDERS

Damage due to alcoholism may be found in any system but the gastrointestinal tract and nervous system are especially at risk.

Acute intoxication

Acute intoxication is usually detectable when the blood level passes 100 mg/100 ml, and is enhanced by barbiturates, benzodiazepines particularly diazepam, chlormethiazole, antidepressants, hypnotics and anticonvulsants, or if the patient's tolerance is reduced by hepatic impairment. The disinhibiting effects of alcohol may lead to hilarity, hostility or maudlin misery. *Manie à potu* is an acute paranoid state with aggression. Cerebellar symptoms of speech and gait develop, then drowsiness. Care must be taken with a comatose patient reeking of alcohol to exclude the complications of head injury, other drugs, gastrointestinal bleeding or hepatic failure.

Alcoholic 'blackouts'

Alcoholic 'blackouts' are gaps of memory covering a period of some hours during which the blood alcohol was above an individual critical level. Memory returns for the 'lost' period at a similar level: an expression of state-dependent learning.

Alcoholic withdrawal states

These often emerge when a regular heavy drinker comes into hospital, for instance for accident surgery, and does not receive his accustomed supplies. The situation may at first mislead the medical team into suspecting a functional psychiatric illness. Increasing tremulousness, sweating, nausea, anxiety and transient hallucinations may start within a few hours of the last drink. Generalised fits may occur within 12-48 hours, with no history of epilepsy. Fits coming on sooner should arise suspicions of head injury or hypoglycaemia, and focal fits demand fuller neurological investigations. Withdrawal fits may be due to bar-biturates or benzodiazepines, especially the short-acting drugs such as lorazepam.

Whatever treatment is given when a diagnosis of alcohol withdrawal has been made — sedation, anticonvulsants or glucose — it is vital to prevent the precipitation of Wernicke's encephalopathy by giving parenteral thiamine, usually in a B and C complex following the manufacturer's instructions.

Delirium tremens is the most dangerous withdrawal state and is usually delayed three to four days. It has the hallmarks of an acute organic brain syndrome with visual, auditory and haptic misinterpreta-tions and hallucinations, fearfulness and nightmares giving way to insomnia. Visual hallucinations are often in miniature. Ceaseless activity, often rehearsing the patient's job, with sweating, tachycardia, fever and dehydration lead to physical exhaustion.

Advice on management may be requested. Skull and chest X-rays are mandatory, and serum electrolytes, urea and glucose must be monitored. Dehydration requires correction, and six litres of fluid daily may be needed. Sedation is essential, and lorazepam is prime choice: both sedating and anticonvulsant, it may be given by any route and, because it is not metabolised in the liver and has a short half-life, it is safer than diazepam or chlormethiazole. Lorazepam may be given in a dosage of 2.5-7.5 mg, four or five times in the 24 hours, for the first 72 hours: just sufficient to control the patient's tremor. After 72 hours the dosage should be progressively reduced so that none is being given on the tenth day. Phenytoin /100 mg up to three times in 24 hours) may also be given if there are fits, and of course parenteral vitamins.

Wernicke-Korsakoff syndrome

Wernicke described a symptomatic triad in 1881: ophthalmoplegia, ataxia and delirium. The encephalopathy, which often presents with part of the triad, is due to acute-on-chronic thiamine deficiency, which can arise in alcoholics and others with gross nutritional deficiency. Treatment is urgent with intravenous thiamine and other vitamins of the B complex and ascorbic acid, followed by daily intramuscular injections for a week. Apart from nystagmus the original symptoms usually subside leaving an amnestic syndrome, Korsakoff psychosis. This is characterised by great difficulty in new learning, from the moment of the insult to the brain, affecting in particular the mamillary bodies. Recall of recent events is thus lost, with preservation of previous memories and other intellectual and social skills. Confabulation is common. Treatment with thiamine is disappointing, but very slow, incomplete improvement occurs with years of abstention.

> *Case*: Mr H., 49, an alcoholic of 25 years' standing, had a delirious episode. Since then he has wept anew every time he is told of his wife's death. Four years later he has begun to say sadly that he believes he may have heard that she had died. His word skills and vocabulary are unscathed.

Alcoholic 'dementia'

Cerebral atrophy and ventricular dilatation develop even before a clinical organic brain syndrome, and both may be reversible over years of abstention. Since the frontal lobes are preferentially involved, judgement, logic and, significantly, self-control are impaired before more tangible indications of brain atrophy. There is no specific treatment.

Alcoholic cerebellar degeneration

This produces a progressively ataxic gait and dysarthria. As in the dementia, toxic rather than nutritional factors are at work: only abstinence helps. Marchiafava-Bignami disease, described first in Italian winos, comprises demyelination of the corpus callosum, causing ataxia, fits, spastic paralysis, dementia and death.

Alcoholic polyneuropathy

Alcoholic polyneuropathy characteristically produces burning, aching and shooting pains in the feet. Thiamine (25-50 mg one to three times daily) or carbamazepine (100 mg twice daily) may help, but seldom; the abstinent course to recovery takes months or years. Retrobulbar neuritis, with dimness of central vision for red and green especially, is a common toxic effect of methyl alcohol, but occasionally occurs with ethanol.

Alcoholic hallucinosis

This may arise while the patient is drinking heavily or in withdrawal. It consists of circumscribed auditory or visual hallucinations, for instance threatening voices or insulting messages written on (bare) walls. Neuroleptics such as trifluoperazine (5-40 mg daily) may be needed for several months. Morbid jealousy is a related condition, and, in both, ideas of reference are common.

Functional psychiatric syndromes

Depression, hypomania or anxiety, especially the latter, may each underlie alcoholic excess, and in turn alcohol abuse may precipitate or exacerbate any of them. Schizophrenic symptoms may also worsen after a drinking episode, and sociopaths commit crimes of violence (Victor, 1983).

MIGRAINE AND OTHER RECURRENT HEADACHES

Acute single episodes of headache are important, but are not the province of the liaison psychiatrist. Occasionally the first attack of migraine, if it involves such neurological symptoms as aphasia, causes alarm. Recurrent, incapacitating headaches are likely to be either migrainous or of the tension type. In the former there is intracranial vasoconstriction preceding extracranial vasodilatation; in the latter there is sustained partial contraction of the muscles of the neck and forehead. Both types are common, recurrent and related to emotional tension.

Migraine

Migraine usually arises in the second and third decades, fading away in the forties and fifties, apart from the infrequent post-menopausal type. There is often a family history of headaches or of allergic disorders, and a personal history of childhood abdominal upsets. The headache of migraine lasts for 8-24 hours and is typically unilateral at its onset and throbbing. Nausea and vomiting usually supervene, with photophobia and noise intolerance. In one-third of cases a visual aura ushers in the attacks, for instance fortification spectra. Variants of migraine include vertebrobasilar, facial, hemiplegic and cluster types (see above). Recognised precipitants may be psychological, dietary including alcohol, fatigue, hypoglycaemia and the contraceptive pill. Migraine sufferers are more often female, and said to be particularly conscientious and perfectionist. In fact no personality type is immune (Henryk-Gutt and Rees, 1973).

Psychological factors seldom operate alone, but it is common for an attack to develop after a period of tension has passed, for instance at the beginning of a vacation or weekend. A wave of irritability anxiety or — less often — pleasant arousal may usher in an attack, and change, during it, to lethargy and depression. Transient disturbances of memory or other cerebral functions may occur. Management of migraine includes realignment of the lifestyle, relaxation training, prophylactics such as pizotifen, clonidine or antidepressants, and in the acute stages simple analgesics, phenergan, or ergotamine if nothing else helps (Lance, 1973, 1976).

Tension headaches

These may occur in patients who also suffer from migraine. The pain is dull and constant: occipital, frontal or like a band round the head. It comes on gradually, especially when the patient is tired; his concentration is poor, and he usually feels tense and stressed during its course as well as at the onset of the headache. Learning factors may apply (Turkat et al., 1984).

Lance (1976) described headaches associated with sexual activity, but more often sexual or other frustration is the forerunner. Relaxation therapy and superficial supportive psychotherapy are more relevant than drugs, but MAOIs sometimes help considerably.

Depressive headache

This is often described in dramatic terms: a weight on top of the head, a feeling of bursting, or like Sydenham's patient a sensation as though a nail were being driven into the head (Sydenham, 1697). Diurnal variations of mood, and symptoms, which include insomnia, loss of appetite and libido, indicate the depressive aetiology. Antidepressants and cognitive manoeuvres are appropriate; MAOIs are usually the most efficacious in depressive and some tension headaches.

In the over-fifties temporal arteritis must be remembered (see above). Persistent post-traumatic headache is considered later with the post-traumatic syndrome.

MOTOR NEURONE DISEASE: AMYOTROPHIC LATERAL SCLEROSIS

This inexorably progressive disease affects, predominantly, men between 50 and 70. Onset is insidious of muscular atrophy with or without spasticity; there are no sensory changes and the sphincters function normally. The combination of upper and lower motor neurone signs is characteristic but diagnostic problems involving the psychiatrist may arise with lesions of the corticospinal tracts above the medulla. These produce loss of emotional control, spastic dysarthria and dysphagia. Despite the hopelessness of his position, it is the relatives rather than the patient who become depressed and resentful and need psychiatric support. Amitriptyline reverses the insulin resistance and impaired glucose utilisation seen in motor neurone disease as in depression, and may reduce muscular fasciculation in the former. It may be worth giving even if the patient shows no overt depression. Doses from 20-80 mg daily or at night are suitable.

POST-TRAUMATIC SYNDROMES

The immediate effects of head injury are a neurosurgical responsibility. After consciousness returns there is a post-traumatic psychosis, lasting minutes to months, and manifesting in any of the symptoms of an organic brain syndrome. These may require psychotropic medication to facilitate nursing and medical management. Post-traumatic (anterograde) and retrograde amnesia are organic effects, but the former is the better guide to severity of brain damage. Both neurological and psychiatric sequelae, particularly the frontal lobe syndrome, are related to the duration of post-traumatic amnesia. Epilepsy is common, and defects of intellect and changes in temperament may be permanent residua of severe head injury. There are pitiably few units — only one in the United Kingdom — where effective behavioural training is available to brain-injured patients whose behaviour rather than intellectual deficit prevents their rehabilitation.

The 'post-traumatic neurosis', so-called, usually follows relatively minor, closed head injury. The definitive work on this subject is Trimble's book (1982). The symptoms of the syndrome are: persistent headache, usually diffuse, and resistant to analgesia; dizziness and light-headedness; anxiety, irritability, restlessness and depression; visual difficulties; poor concentration and low confidence.

Aggravating factors include work, worry, noise, eye strain and domestic pressures. Other factors affecting outcome are premorbid personality, emotional impact of the injury, social and career implications, legal and compensation issues, and personal support system (Tarsh and Royston, 1985).

Case: Mr M.J., 46, returned from Australia with his wife and two children, having failed to find a good job there. On the way to a possible post in Britain he was involved in a road traffic accident, for which he was not to blame. Although he was not concussed, two years later he still suffers from headaches and visual disturbances for which no physical cause has been identified, but which prevent his working as a waiter. He is tense and irritable, and a legal case is pending.

In 1961 the forthright neurologist Henry Miller reported a follow-up study of patients with psychoneurotic symptoms after head injury. Forty-five out of 50 re-examined two years after settlement of their compensation claims had recovered, implying a mixed aetiology for their symptoms (Miller, 1961). It seems plausible that head injury, like other insults involving the brain, may disrupt neurotransmitter activity, and lead to a neurotic reaction to a minor neurological upset. Malingering is extremely rare.

Very occasionally small doses of major or minor tranquillisers will cut short the post-traumatic neurosis in its early stages. More often it is fruitless — despite colleagues' pressure — to treat the patient before the lawyers are done, unless he is really keen to receive treatment. Most patients do well, at the appropriate time, on a tranylcypromine (10 mg) and trifluoperazine (1 mg) combination, as in the case of Mr M.J. Two or three doses daily, before 4 pm, are usually sufficient.

REFERENCES AND FURTHER READING

Bagley, C. (1972) 'Social Prejudice and the Adjustment of People with Epilepsy', *Epilepsia, 13*, 33-45

Bear, D.M. and Fedio, P. (1977) 'Qualitative Analysis of Interictal Behaviour in Temporal Lobe Epilepsy', *Archives of Neurology, 34*, 454-67

Beard, A.W. and Slater, E. (1962) 'The Schizophrenia-like Psychoses of Epilepsy', *Proceedings of the Royal Society of Medicine, 55*, 311-16

Beccle, H.C. (1946) *Psychiatry*, Faber, London

British Medical Journal (1981) Leader, 'Levodopa: Long-term Impact in Parkinson's Disease', *British Medical Journal, 282*, 417

Buchsbaum, M.S., Ingvar, D.H., Kessler, R., Waters, R.N., Cappelletti, J., van Kammen, D.P., King, A.C., Johnson, J.L., Manning, R.C., Flynn, R.W., Mann, L.S., Bunneym W.E. and Sokologg, L. (1982) 'Cerebral Glycography with Positron Tomography', *Archives of General Psychiatry, 39*, 251-9

Caine, E.C. and Shoulson, I. (1983) 'Psychiatric Syndromes in Huntington's Disease', *American Journal of Psychiatry, 140*, 728-33

Charcot, J.M. (1877) *Lectures on Diseases of the Nervous System* (translated by Siegerson, G.), New Sydenham Society, London

Cutting, H. (1983) 'Acute Organic Reactions', in Lader, M.H. (Ed.) *'Mental Disorders and Somatic Illness'*, Cambridge University Press, Cambridge

De Paulo, J.R. and Folstein, M.F. (1978) 'Psychiatric Disturbances in Neurological Patients; Detection, Recognition and Hospital Course', *Annals of Neurology, 4*, 225-8

Dewhurst, K. (1969) 'The Neurosyphilitic Psychosis Today', *British Journal of Psychiatry, 115*, 31-8

Dewhurst, K. (1970) 'Personality Disorders in Huntington's Disease', *Psychiatrica Clinica, 3*, 221-9

Fenton, G.W. (1983) 'Epilepsy', in Lader, M.H. (Ed.) *Mental Disorders and Somatic Illness*, Cambridge University Press, Cambridge

Flor-Henry, P. (1969) 'Schizophrenia-like Reactions and Affective Psychoses Associated with Temporal Lobe Epilepsy: Aetiological Factors', *American Journal of Psychiatry, 126*, 400-4

Folstein, M.F. and McHugh, P.R. (1983) 'The Neuropsychiatry of Some Specific Brain Disorders', in Lader, M.H. (Ed.) *Mental Disorders and Somatic Illness*, Cambridge University Press, Cambridge

Folstein, M.F., Maiberger, R. and McHugh, P.R. (1977) 'Mood Disorders as a Complication of Stroke', *Journal of Neurology, Neurosurgery and Psychiatry, 40*, 1018-20

Gomez, J. (1985) 'Psychological Aspects of Pain', paper presented at conference on the Pharmacology of Pain, Cardiff

Harper, P.S. (1983) 'A Genetic Marker for Huntington's Chorea', *British Medical Journal, 287*, 1567-8

Hawton, K., Fagg, J. and Marsack, D. (1980) 'Association between Epilepsy and Attempted Suicide', *Journal of Neurology, Neurosurgery and Psychiatry, 43*, 148-70

Henryk-Gutt, R. and Rees, W.L. (1973) 'Psychological Aspects of Migraine', *Journal of Psychosomatic Research, 17*, 141-53

Kahana, E., Lebowitz, W. and Alter, M. (1971) 'Cerebral Multiple Sclerosis', *Neurology, 21*, 1179-85

Kirk, C. and Saunders, H. (1977) 'Primary Psychiatric Illness in a Neurological Outpatient Department in North East England', *Acta Psychiatrica Scandinavica, 56*, 294-302

Koehler, K. and Sass, H. (1984) 'Affective Psychopathology in Huntington's Disease', *Psychological Medicine, 14*, 733-7

Lance, J.W. (1973) *The Mechanism and Management of Headache*, 2nd Edition, Butterworths, London

Lance, J.W. (1976) 'Headache', *British Journal of Hospital Medicine, 19*, 377-9

Lipowski, Z.J. and Kiriakos, R. (1972) 'Borderlands between Neurology and Psychiatry: Observations in a Neurological Hospital', *Psychiatry in Medicine, 3*, 131-47

Lishman, W.A. (1978) *Organic Psychiatry*, Blackwell, London

Miller, H. (1961) 'Accident Neurosis', *British Medical Journal, 1*, 919-25

Perez, M.H., Trimble, M.R., Murray, N.M.F. and Reider, I. (1985) 'Epileptic Psychosis: an Evaluation of P.S.E. Profiles', *British Journal of Psychiatry, 146*, 155-63

Pond, D.A. (1957) 'Psychiatric Aspects of Epilepsy', *Journal of the Indian Medical Profession, 3*, 1441-51

Reil, J.C. (1808) 'Research upon the Method of Cure in Mental Disorders', quoted in Hunter, R. and Macalpine, I. (1963) *Three Hundred Years of Psychiatry*, Oxford University Press, London

Ridley, R.M., Baker, H.F. and Crow, T.J. (1986) 'Transmissible and Non-transmissible Neurodegenerative Disease', *Psychological Medicine, 16*, 188-208

Roberts, J.K.A. (1984) *Differential Diagnosis in Neuropsychiatry*, Wiley, London and New York

Roy, A. (1977) 'Hysterical Fits Previously Diagnosed as Epilepsy', *Psychological Medicine, 7*, 271-3

Rutter, M., Graham, P.J. and Yule, W. (1970) 'A Neuropsychiatric Study in Childhood', *Clinics in Developmental Medicine*, Heinemann, London

Saugstad, L. and Odegard, O. (1986) 'Huntington's Chorea in Norway', *Psychological Medicine, 16*, 39-48

Scott, D.F. (1978) 'Psychiatric Aspects of Epilepsy', *British Journal of Psychiatry, 132*, 417-30

Slater, E. and Glithero, E. (1965) 'A Follow-up of Patients Diagnosed as Suffering from Hysteria', *Journal of Psychosomatic Research, 9*, 9-13

Stores, G. (1978) 'School Children with Epilepsy at Risk for Learning and Behaviour Problems', *Developmental Medicine and Child Neurology, 20*, 505-8

Storey, P.B. (1972) 'Emotional Disablement before and after Subarachnoid Haemorrhage', in *Physiology, Emotion and Psychosomatic Illness*, Ciba Foundation Symposium. Elsevier, Amsterdam

Surridge, D. (1969) 'An Investigation into Some Psychiatric Aspects of Multiple Sclerosis', *British Journal of Psychiatry, 115*, 749-64

Sydenham, T. (1697) 'Discourse Concerning Hysterical Passion', in *Dr Sydenham's Complete Method of Curing Almost All Diseases*, 3rd edition, Cave, London

Tarsh, M.J. and Royston, C. (1985) 'A Follow-up Study of Accident Neurosis', *British Journal of Psychiatry, 146*, 18-25

Toone, B.K. (1980) Personal Communication quoted by Fenton, G.N. in Chapter 13, Lader, M.H. (Ed.) *Mental Disorders and Somatic Illness*, (1983), Cambridge University Press, Cambridge

Toone, B.K., Wheeler, M. and Fenwick, P.B.C. (1980) 'Sex Hormone Changes in Male Epileptics', *Endocrinology, 12*, 391-5

Tramont, E.C. (1979) '*Treponema pallidum*', in Mandell, G.L., Douglas, R.G. and Bennett, J.G. (Eds) *Principle and Practice of Infectious Diseases*, Wiley, New York

Trimble, M.R. (1981) *Neuropsychiatry*, Wiley, Chichester and New York

Trimble, M.R. (1982) *Post-traumatic Neurosis*, Wiley, Chichester and New York

Turkat, I.D. Kuczmierczyk, A.R. and Adams, H.E. (1984) 'An Investigation of the Aetiology of Chronic Headache: the Role of Headache Models', *British Journal of Psychiatry, 145*, 665-6

Victor, M. (1983) 'Mental Disorders due to Alcoholism' in Lader, M.H. (Ed.) *Mental Disorders and Somatic Illness*, Cambridge University Press, Cambridge

von Meduna, L. (1937) *Die Konvulsiontherapie der Schizophrenie*, Halle, Marburg

Walton, J.M. (1974) *Essentials of Neurology*, 4th edition, Pitman Medical, London

Wernicke, C. (1881) *Lehrbuch der Gehirnkrankheiten für Aetze und Studirende*, Fischer, Kassel

Whitlock, F.A. (1977) 'Depression and Suicide', in Burrows, G.D. (Ed.) *Handbook on Studies in Depression*, Elsevier, Amsterdam

Whitlock, F.A. (1982) Chapters 5 and 6, in *Symptomatic Affective Disorders*, Academic Press, Sydney

Wolf, P. and Trimble, M.R., (1985) 'Biological Antagonism and Epileptic Psychosis', *British Journal of Psychiatry, 146*, 272-6

6

Liaison in Cardiorespiratory Disorders

Emotional states are reflected and expressed through changes in cardiorespiratory function. The heart is the organ of love in every language. It beats faster with sexual excitement, hope, fear and rage. The dejected are heavy-hearted. Laughing and weeping are respiratory behaviours; we 'hold our breath' in peril, feel suffocated in anxiety and respond by hyperventilation. Influenced as it may be by the emotional climate, the efficient operation of the cardiovascular and respiratory apparatus is urgently necessary for survival. More Americans and Europeans die from acute or chronic cardiorespiratory dysfunction than from any other cause (Knowles, 1977). Because of advances in the medical treatment of infection, and the ageing of the population, the chronic diseases are increasingly prevalent — and important. They are partly, at least, the results of lifestyle, including: emotional stress, tobacco and other pollution, alcohol, over-nourishment, too little physical activity and central heating.

HYPERTENSION

High blood pressure is probably the biggest single risk factor for morbidity and mortality in the West, significant in the causation of both coronary heart disease and stroke. It affects up to 20 per cent of the population (Matarazzo, 1982), even on the over-strict criteria of the World Health Organization of 1959: arterial blood pressure persistently higher than 140-160/90-95. Essential hypertension embraces the 80-90 per cent of cases without obvious organic aetiology, such as renal impairment, adrenal disturbance or coarctation of the aorta.

The liaison psychiatrist is involved from two angles: to disentangle psychoneurotic, iatrogenic and organic factors in symptomatology, and to advise on management and prophylaxis in this potentially lethal condition.

Uncomplicated hypertension is essentially symptomless, and before diagnosis those patients who turn out to have a raised blood pressure come over as being particularly stable and free of complaint (Herrmann *et al.*, 1976). Recognised hypertensives, however, may report a multiplicity of symptoms, which they understandably attribute to their abnormal blood pressure or to medical treatment. Tiredness and exhaustion, reduced sexual interest and sleepiness occur in 70 per cent; headaches, unsteadiness, depressed mood, weak limbs, dry mouth and palpitations in 40-45 per cent; and vivid dreams, vertigo, insomnia, gastrointestinal dysfunction, impotence and ejaculatory difficulty in up to 20 per cent. The characteristic symptom complexes for depression and anxiety derived from questionnaires such as the General Health Questionnaire and the Middlesex Hospital Questionnaire, and from semi-structured interviews are found in 60 per cent of diagnosed hypertensives. These psychoneurotic manifestations correlate significantly with most of the other symptoms. The exceptions are undue fatigue, gastrointestinal problems and practical sexual difficulties in men (Bulpitt *et al.*, 1977; Mann, 1984).

The possible undesirable effects of hypotensive medication

The intended lowering of the blood pressure may overshoot, and even if it is only reduced to a normal level, initially at any rate, the patient may feel tired, drowsy and weak. Unwanted side-effects are erectile and ejaculatory failure in men, postural hypotension, dry mouth, blurred vision and depression. Methyldopa has a central action analogous to that of the *Rauwolfia* alkaloids, depleting the brain of monoamine transmitters: the result may be to bring forward a depressive episode of the endogenous type in those susceptible. Beta-blockers act competitively at beta-adrenoreceptor sites and may lead to depression by their central effects; atenolol has less central effect than others such as propanolol. Clonidine has mixed central and peripheral actions and has also been associated with depression. Guanethidine and related postganglionic sympathetic blockers have no demonstrable central effects but may prevent ejaculation and cause impotence, with secondary depression in some men. Thiazide diuretics have no direct influence on mood.

When a hypertensive patient is clinically depressed, it must be remembered that tricycle antidepressants cancel part of the effectiveness of the guanethidine group and also of clonidine. MAOIs are in themselves hypotensive and particularly suitable for the combined tension and depression common in hypertensives. However, they interact dangerously with methyldopa and potentiate the hypotensive effects of sympathetic blockers, and the 'cheese reaction' is especially undesirable in a hypertensive. Trazodone and mianserin are safe choices of antidepressants in relation to hypotensive agents, but may make the patient feel even more lethargic (Bulpitt and Dollery, 1973; Lishman, 1978; Morgan, 1983). Trazodone is given in a dosage of 100-300 mg, divided, in 24 hours.

In Mann's account (1984) of the large Medical Research Council study, improvement in psychologically mediated symptoms, independently of changes in blood pressure, was shown to be due to the ongoing interest and support accorded to this cohort of patients. Non-pharmacological manoeuvres are of value for the blood pressure itself, in the management of obesity which is a major adverse factor in some cases, and in reducing psychological distress. Biofeedback, and relaxation therapies both group and individual, give the patient the satisfaction of participating in his treatment.

Prophylactic measures

The long-held view that hypertension results from repressed hostility (Alexander, 1939; Groen *et al.*, 1971) has received a setback from Mann's study using the Hostility and Direction of Hostility Questionnaire (Mann, 1977). Hypertensive patients compared with normotensives showed a trend to higher scores on the scales for outwardly directed criticism and acting out hostility; but questionnaires in psychiatry may miss the subtleties of unconscious mental mechanisms. A persistent elevation of blood pressure has been demonstrated in various situations of stress and helplessness in some people. Symptomless increase in blood pressure was shown to occur in 27 per cent of soldiers after a year on active service (Graham, 1945), or, more relevant today, in men awaiting redundancy (Kasl and Cobb, 1970). Known hypertensives and, less understandably, their close associates whether or not blood relatives, respond to events more than other people by a rise in arterial pressure. Psychotherapy for patients and their families should focus on safer ways of adapting to stressful situations.

Complications

Cardiac effects may be reflected in shortness of breath, angina or swollen ankles. If the cerebral vasculature takes the brunt, neurological or mental symptoms arise: transiently, with a single stroke, or in little steps. Dulling of intellect, personality and memory, often with depression and enhancement of paranoid traits, may result from multiple minor ischaemic episodes.

Modern treatment of hypertension has made the malignant phase a rarity, but occasionally very high pressures present with severe headache and visual failure. Hypertensive encephalopathy is a medical emergency, developing rapidly with headache, drowsiness, apprehension and confusion. Vomiting and papilloedema indicate raised intracranial pressure, and there is always retinopathy. Cardiac and renal functions are compromised, and without urgent treatment coma leads on to death. The pathology comprises cerebral oedema, petechial haemorrhages and micro-infarcts.

ISCHAEMIC HEART DISEASE (IHD)

A coronary attack is aptly called the Western way of death. More patients are surviving myocardial infarction, presenting physicians and psychiatrists with the challenge of reversing a life pattern that leads to disaster, often at the peak time in a man's progress when his employer and his family value him most. The precursors of a first — or a subsequent — infarction are multifactorial: raised blood lipid levels, associated with high fat intake, myxoedema or diabetes mellitus; hypertension; obesity; smoking; physical underactivity; and pyknic build.

Type A behaviour

William Osler (1928) first described the Type A man as a typical angina pectoris patient: 'the robust, the vigorous in mind and body, the keen and ambitious man, the indicator of whose engine is always full speed ahead'. Friedman and Rosenman (1959) demonstrated the dangers of coronary-prone behaviour. It is associated with increased atheroma, increased diurnal secretion of adrenalin involving greater myocardial oxygen requirement, increased numbers of ectopic beats and raised heart rate when under ego threat. Type A characteristics are an exaggerated sense of time urgency, excessive competitiveness and striving for achievement, and hostility and aggressiveness: the qualities appreciated by the modern employer.

With these qualities and one or more of the other risk factors a man, or less often a woman, is set to develop angina or have a sudden overt or silent coronary in response to a major life event (Bayliss, 1985: Connolly, 1985).

Angina

Left-sided chest pain, perhaps radiating to arm or jaw, may be associated with disturbance of myocardial function, usually ischaemic: the harbinger of heart attack to come. It is also a common symptom of anxiety and, less often, of depression. Bass and Wade (1984) studied 99 patients admitted with chest pain and presumptive IHD. Fifty-three had significant heart disease and the others a form of neurosis. It was the latter who had most complaints of breathlessness at rest, palpitations, faintness, giddiness and a feeling of suffocation; in just as many their symptoms had lasted five years or more. These anxious cardioneurotic patients are the modern equivalent of sufferers from da Costa's syndrome, effort syndrome, soldier's heart and 'betahyperresponsiveness', reviewed by Skerritt (1983).

Post-myocardial infarction

Most patients respond well to the impact of heart attack, passing through a stage of denial to one of constructive realism. Eighty-five per cent are working a year later, not necessarily in the same job, although the frequency of sexual activity may remain reduced indefinitely. The patients who do not pick up the threads of their lives become irritable, touchy and depressed, and are in danger of dependent cardiac invalidism.

Predictive factors for a poor outcome

These include manual work, and severe cardiological symptoms; an anxious, overprotective spouse; no spouse; poor premorbid adjustment, maritally, socially and at work (Mayou, 1984).

Therapeutic support

At-risk patients and those overtly depressed need intensive encourage-ment from the whole therapeutic team, and family therapy. Educa-tional and group psychotherapeutic support is of no particular benefit to the general run of post-coronary patients, but Patel *et al.* (1985) report a useful outcome, on four-year follow up, of an eight-week course of relaxation therapy. The methods they use include medita-tion, breathing exercises and instruction in managing stress. Reduc-tion in diastolic and systolic pressures, fewer electrocardiographic abnormalities and complaints of angina arose in the patients given relaxation compared with controls.

CARDIAC SURGERY

Post-cardiotomy delirium affects 25-50 per cent of patients, usually coming on three to five days after surgery and lasting three to five days. 'Emergence delirium', a transient post-anaesthetic confusional state, is less important. The major delirium often requires treatment with haloperidol for five days and the general treatment for acute brain syndromes (Chapter 3). Sometimes a state of irritability and paranoia persists for a week or two, and small doses of the neuroleptic (1.5 mg twice daily) should continue. Predisposing factors are age, cerebral impairment, severe social and marital problems, and marked preoperative anxiety. The latter should be sought and ameliorated by discussion, reassurance and benzodiazepines (Morse, 1976; Lipowski, 1980). Postoperative depressive reactions are also more likely in those showing anxiety earlier. In all postoperative psychological upset, the patient's metabolic state, hydration and drug status need checking.

ACUTE RESPIRATORY INFECTIONS

These comprise acute bronchitis, bacterial pneumonia and viral pneumonia including influenzal. Any of them may cause hypoxia and a confusional state, but the most florid symptoms, with plucking of the bedclothes, disorientation, hallucinations and gross misinterpreta-tions, occur in pneumococcal pneumonia. Delirium comes on over a matter of hours and lasts for two to ten days: it may be enhanced by alcohol or drug withdrawal, cerebral impairment or cardiac insuf-ficiency. It is important not to mistake an acute or subacute organic brain syndrome for dementia in the elderly or for schizophrenia in the comparatively young: see Chapter 3 for details and management. Pneumonia is particularly likely to affect the very old and very young, alcoholics, vagrants, and those immobilised for any reason. It is sometimes the presenting complaint of an unrecognised myocardial infarction.

Whereas acute organic psychosis at the height of the infection is the major psychiatric concern in most severe respiratory illness, with influenza the impact is more often affective, and comes in the convalescent phase. Tuke in 1892 described 15 post-influenzal cases: eleven depressed, four manic. More recently Whitlock (1982) wrote of 'a spate of depression', sometimes suicidal, following influenza. Understanding, emotional support and a tricyclic antidepressant are indicated, with follow-up for three months or more.

BRONCHIAL ASTHMA

Aretaeus saw this as a psychosomatic disorder as far back as the second century. Neurogenic imbalance, allergic reactions and psychological influences all operate. Mucosal hyperfunction, essential to an attack, results from vagal stimulation however set off; spasm of the bronchial musculature is analogous in its multifactorial mechanism to the spasms of irritable colon; and habitual abnormal breathing patterns compress the larger bronchi, making it difficult to exhale — but easier with the lips part closed (Groen, 1976). Asthmatic attacks are often precipitated by an intense emotional experience: perhaps sexual, or a quarrel, in competitive sport, or — for a child — at his birthday party. Alexander *et al.* (1968) believed that the underlying cause is a conflict between feeling fear or anger and dependency, so that verbal expression is inhibited. Certainly non-verbal behaviours such as laughing or crying may set off an attack; so may physical or mental exertion, involving — perhaps — unspoken feelings.

Operant conditioning

Parents, teachers, friends and spouses may inadvertently reinforce asthmatic behaviour, for example by excusing the patient from something he dislikes or fears if he begins to wheeze. This applies to sexual intercourse, examinations, playing bridge, or housework, and there is also the secondary gain of sympathy and concern.

Management

The advice of the liaison psychiatrist makes a valuable addition to the physician's treatment package. Children with asthma form a special group, and the avoidance of operant conditioning is particularly important for them. Children with asthma may be allergic to the housedust mite, but there are likely to be conflicting reasons also for the common experience that attacks diminish if a child goes into hospital, or away to school. Growing up, for various reasons, means leaving childhood asthma behind in up to 78 per cent of cases (including that of Charles Dickens). Helping an adolescent to separate emotionally from mother — and father — may complete the cure.

It is significant that, among older asthmatics, placebos and suggestion reduce the number of attacks in both atopic and non-atopic asthma. Breathing exercises increase confidence and correct maladaptive respiratory responses. Biofeedback, behavioural manoeuvres, desensitising the patient to situations that provoke attacks, relaxation and autohypnosis: all are effective in some patients. Psychotherapy, particularly in groups, couples and family may release underlying conflicts and misinterpretations, so that they may be dealt with. Learning to recognise the onset of a genuine attack, by the use of a de Bono whistle, helps patients to use their medication efficiently: 'feeling dreadful' is not a reliable warning of respiratory malfunction, and vice versa. A curious anomaly for a disorder associated with emotional tension is the reported rarity of asthmatic attacks in concentration camps (Groen, 1976).

CHRONIC OBSTRUCTIVE AIRWAYS DISEASE (COAD)

Chronic bronchitis, emphysema and chronic asthma are incapacitating, alarming and depressing; thoughts of death often precede respiratory failure. The course of the illness is a slow decline studded with exacerbations, and more or less hypoxia. Psychiatric associations include: anxiety and depression, both of which make the symptoms worse; depression, hypochondriasis; paranoid states; sexual incapacity; alcoholism and tobacco addiction.

Psychiatric aspects of management

Psychotropic medication

Benzodiazepine anxiolytics depress respiration and are anyway a poor substitute for education and psychotherapy, except, occasionally, with a panic attack. Antidepressants such as doxepin, amitriptyline or maprotiline are immediately effective in reducing anxiety and insomnia, but take a week or more to have an impact on depression. Tricyclic antidepressants are compatible with bronchodilators and potentiate the steroids often prescribed in COAD. If dry mouth and thick mucus are troublesome the best tricyclic is desipramine. For all the tricyclics just mentioned a daily dosage, divided or at night, ranges from 50-200 mg. Among the neuroleptics, haloperidol is generally suitable, for its lower peripheral autonomic effects. Dosage should be kept down to 3-15 mg in 24 hours if possible. It may be needed in the COAD patient who develops an acute organic brain syndrome, a paranoid state, agitation in either depression or dementia, or mania. The latter may crop up in reaction to corticosteroids or coincidentally.

Psychological/psychotherapeutic approaches

The aims are to maximise psychosocial support, so that the patient feels cared for and respected; to train him in coping skills, that is, realistic problem-solving; and to encourage his adaptive abilities, that is, changes within himself, and finding new sources of gratification. It is important that one therapist, or the team, should establish a supporting relationship with the patient, not only during crises, and encourage him to express his feelings without fear of criticism or unwanted probing (Petrich and Holmes, 1980). Breathing exercises, relaxation and physical activity progammes may keep patients going for longer. Group therapy is likely to be most helpful if it is physically oriented or supportive: those with COAD are harmed rather than helped by interpretive group therapy (Rosser *et al.*, *1983*).

BRONCHIAL CARCINOMA

The liaison aspects of oncology and of terminal illness are dealt with in Chapters 13 and 14 respectively. Lung cancer often develops in a bronchitic patient, and is particularly likely to be preceded by depression. Cerebral secondaries are also common in this cancer, and manifest in visual, neurological or psychiatric symptoms, occasionally as the first presentation of the disease. Cushingoid effects including affective symptoms, mainly depressive, may be seen in ACTH-producing tumours of the lung.

Sarcoid carcinoma, though less serious, has features in common with bronchial carcinoma: the patient is fatigued and often depressed, and cerebral sarcoid may produce neuropsychiatric symptoms.

HYPERVENTILATION SYNDROME

Fast, shallow breathing is part of a normal autonomic response to anxiety-provoking situations; it may also occur with phobic or free-floating anxiety. Hyperventilation is usually short-lived and occurs only occasionally. Some subjects, particularly those of perfectionist personality who are irritated or made anxious more readily than most, are habitual hyperventilators. They may induce various alarming symptoms in themselves which in turn provoke concern. Washing out arterial carbon dioxide makes the neurones alkaline, leading to hyper-irritability — and even fits, tremor, spasms and paraesthesiae. Parasympathetic depression produces relative sympathetic overactivity: tachycardia, palpitations, irritability of gut and bladder and excessive sweating. Hypoxia may manifest in dizziness and altered consciousness (Pincus, 1978, Kraft and Hooguin, 1984). If hyperventilation can be demonstrated to bring on the symptoms that worry the patient, it is worth while to apply the Papworth technique involving breathing exercises and relaxation in co-ordination (Cluff, 1984).

REFERENCES

Alexander, F. (1939) 'Emotional Factors in Arterial Hypertension', *Psychosomatic Medicine, 1*, 175-9

Alexander, F., French, T.M. and Pollock, G. (1968) *Psychosomatic Specificity*, University of Chicago Press, Chicago

Bass, C. and Wade, C. (1984) 'Chest Pain with Normal Coronary Arteries: a Comparative Study of Psychiatric and Social Morbidity', *Psychological Medicine, 14*, 51-61.

Bayliss, R.I.S. (1985) 'The Silent Coronary', *British Medical Journal, 290*, 1093-4

Bulpitt, C.J. and Dollery, C.T. (1973) 'Side Effects of Hypotensive Agents Evaluated by a Self-administered Questionnaire', *British Medical Journal, 3*, 485-90

Bulpitt, C.J., Dollery, C.T. and Hoffbrand, B.I. (1977) 'The Contribution of Psychological Features to the Symptoms of Treated Hypertensive

Patients', *Psychological Medicine, 7*, 661-5

Cluff, R.A. (1984) 'Chronic Hyperventilation and its Treatment by Physiotherapy, a Discussion Paper', *Journal of the Royal Society of Medicine, 77*, 855-62

Connolly, J. (1985) 'Life's Happenings and Organic Disease', *British Journal of Hospital Medicine, 33*, 24-7

Friedman, M. and Rosenman, R.H. (1959) 'Association of Specific Overt Behaviour Patterns with Blood and Cardiovascular Findings', *Journal of the American Medical Association, 169*, 1286-96

Graham, J.D.P. (1945) 'High Blood Pressure after Battle', *Lancet, 1*, 239-40

Groen, J.J. (1976) Chapter 12 in Hill, O.W. (Ed.), *Modern Trends in Psychosomatic Medicine — 3*, Butterworths, London

Groen, J.J., van der Valk, J.M. and Weiner, A. (1971) 'Psychological Factors in the Pathogenesis of Essential Hypertension', *Psychotherapy and Psychosomatics, 19*, 1-26

Herrmann, H.J.M., Rassek, M., Schafer, N., Schmidt, Th. and Von Uexkull, Th. (1976) Chapter 13 in Hill, O.W. (Ed.), *Modern Trends in Psychosomatic Medicine — 3* , Butterworths, London

Kasl, S.V. and Cobb, S. (1970) 'Blood Pressure Changes in Men Undergoing Job Loss: a Preliminary Report', *Psychosomatic Medicine, 32*, 19-38

Knowles, J. (1977) 'The Responsibility of the Individual', in Knowles, J. (Ed.) *Doing Better and Feeling Worse: Health in the United States*, Norton, New York

Kraft, A.R. and Hooguin, C.A.L. (1984) 'The Hyperventilation Syndrome: a Pilot Study on the Effectiveness of Treatment', *British Journal of Psychiatry, 145*, 538-42

Lipowski, Z.J. (1980) 'Delirium in Surgery', *Delirium, Acute Brain Failure in Man*, Thomas, Springfield, Ill.

Lishman, W.A. (1978) Chapter 9, *Organic Psychiatry*, Blackwell, Oxford

Mann, A. (1977) 'Psychiatric Morbidity and Hostility in Hypertension', *Psychological Medicine, 7*, 653-9

Mann, A. (1984) 'Hypertension: Psychological Aspects and Diagnostic Impact in a Clinical Trial', *Monograph Supplement 5; Psychological Medicine*, Cambridge University Press, Cambridge

Matarazzo, J.D. (1982) 'Behavioural Health's Challenge to Academic, Scientific and Professional Psychology', *American Psychologist, 37*, 1-14

Mayou, R. (1984) 'Prediction of Emotional and Social Outcome after a Heart Attack', *Journal of Psychosomatic Research, 28*, 17-25

Morgan, H.G. (1983) Chapter 2, in Lader, M.H. (Ed.) *Mental Disorders and Somatic Illness*, Cambridge University Press, Cambridge

Morse, R.M. (1976) 'Psychiatry and Surgical Delirium', in Howells, J.G. (Ed.) *Modern Trends in Psychosomatic Medicine — 3*, Butterworths, London

Osler, W. (1928) *Principles and Practice of Medicine*, Appleton-Century-Crofts, New York

Patel, C., Marmot, M.G., Terry, D.J., Carruthers, M., Hunt, B. and Patel, M. (1985) 'Trial of Relaxation in Reducing Coronary Risk: Four-year Follow up', *British Medical Journal, 290*, 1103-6

Petrich. J. and Holmes, T.H. (1980) Chapter 11, in Hall, R.C.W. (Ed.), *Psychiatric Presentations of Physical Illness*, Spectrum, New York

Pincus, J.H. (1978) 'Hyperventilation Syndrome', *British Journal of Hospital Medicine, 19*, 312-13

Rosser, R., Denford, J., Heslop, A., Kinston, W., Macklin, D., Minty, K., Moynihan, C., Muir, B., Rein, L. and Guz, A. (1984) 'Breathlessness and Psychiatric Morbidity in Chronic Bronchitis and Emphysema: a Study of Psychotherapeutic Management', *Psychological Medicine, 13*, 93-110

Skerritt, P.W. (1983) 'Anxiety and the Heart', *Psychological Medicine, 13*, 17-25

Tuke, G.H. (1892) *Dictionary of Psychological Medicine*, Churchill, London

Whitlock, F.A. (1982) Chapter 2, in *Symptomatic Affective Disorders*, Academic Press, Sydney

7

Liaison in Gastrointestinal Problems

Emotions and relationships with others are intimately linked with gastrointestinal function from birth. The first nutritional experience involves close association with mother who may be anxious, excited, elated or exhausted. Although feeding and meal times remain central in human concourse, there is a significant period when a major focus of interest in relation to important others, particularly mother, is elimination and its control. Concepts of naughtiness, dirtiness and disgust are driven home during this phase. To feel soiled or contaminated is always distressing and humiliating. One feature of dying most feared, particularly with gastrointestinal patients, is the possibility of losing eliminatory control.

Different functions have contrasting symbolic meanings. Sharing food equates with sharing life; elimination implies rejection from fear, anger or revulsion: 'He makes me sick', 'He's a shit.'

ABDOMINAL PAIN

Acute pain demands acute surgical or medical measures. In children with chronic or recurrent abdominal pain severe enough to warrant specialist opinion, the underlying pathology in more than 90 per cent is primarily psychiatric. Disturbed family relationships or stresses from changes at school are commonly found, and in those children who are emotionally insecure may set off gastrointestinal symptoms, perhaps through gastric hyperaemia or increased gut motility. Obvious organic disorders must be excluded, including fashionable lactose and other food intolerance, but extensive investigations are counterproductive: the child psychiatrist should take over. About one-quarter of these children continue suffering abdominal pain for years and even into adult life (Nichol, 1982).

Adults with non-acute abdominal pain are also surprisingly likely to have a psychological rather than an organic disorder. In a study of 96 cases referred by their general practitioners to a surgical or a medical gastroenterology clinic because of pain, only 15 were considered to have physical disease. Twelve drank excessively and may have suffered transient episodes of gastritis, and of the remaining 69, 32 were clinically depressed, 21 had chronic tension states, and 17 owed their symptoms to hysterical conversion. In follow-up over seven years one patient developed endometriosis and one man who had taken an overdose was found to have a colonic carcinoma (Gomez and Dally, 1977). It is regrettable that liaison is seldom requested at the outpatient stage for adults with abdominal pain, since it would clearly be of benefit to these patients (especially women, who have significantly more psychologically-mediated abdominal pain: (Gomez and Dally, 1977) in whom organic pathology is doubtful, to have a psychiatric assessment and therapy options (See Chapter 4). Often an opinion is requested after surgery if symptoms fail to subside (Gomez, 1984).

SPECIFIC GASTROINTESTINAL DISORDERS

Peptic ulcer

Peptic ulcer has been considered the paradigm of psychosomatic disease. In fact several disparate disorders come under this head. The typical acute gastroduodenal ulcer is the 'stress ulcer' which arises after major trauma, especially head injury, cerebral surgery, burns, sepsis, renal failure, and the ingestion of corticosteroids or aspirin. It varies in site and presentation according to causation (Wangensteen and Golden, 1973). Hyperparathyroidism may also lead to gastric ulcer, accompanied by such psychiatric manifestations as anxiety or psychosis (see Chapter 9).

Chronic ulceration may be either gastric or duodenal. The former tends to affect older patients and carries a 10 per cent risk of malignancy. Those whose ulcers develop on the lesser curvature of the stomach are a genetically separate group, belonging to blood group A rather than O and with differing secretion of gastric acid: much more or less than the norm (Ackerman and Weiner, 1976). High serum pepsinogen levels predispose to duodenal disease (Mirsky, 1958). For the development of psychosomatic disease in general, requirements in varying degree are organic susceptibility (in this case high pepsinogen and low mucosal resistance), emotional stress or conflict, and adverse environmental factors. It used to be thought that stresses of

112

business were a sure route to duodenal ulceration, but today the type A, go-getting executive is said to be coronary rather than ulcer prone. Nevertheless, continued or recurrent conflict may lead, in the vulnerable, to duodenal ulcer. Cigarette-smoking and regular dosage of alcohol offer spurious relief to those under pressure, and are common currency in the world of commerce — one reason why men are affected by duodenal ulcer four times as often as women.

Ulcer-type pain may recur after an ulcer has healed, or arise without ulcer as symptom of tension or depression or an hysterical escape mechanism in a demanding situation. In either case psychotherapy helps in explanation and by facilitating realistic adjustments in lifestyle, smoother methods of coping with insecurity personally and at work, better use of relationships, and a shift in attitude towards conservation rather than exploitation of self. It is often necessary to use medication, for instance phenelzine, to ameliorate both tension and abdominal symptoms before useful discussions can be held.

Case: Mr G.T., a tube-train driver of 49, developed persistent ulcer-type symptoms when there was a major disaster on another underground line coinciding with a personal upset: his first grandchild was born with spina bifida. He improved with an MAOI and support, and encouragement to spend more time on his hobby of painting by numbers. He did well apart from a temporary relapse when a second grandchild was expected.

Cimetidine and to a lesser extent ranitidine, while excellent in procuring ulcer healing, sometimes induce impotence as a side-effect and/or depression. It is worth remembering, however, that recovery from his duodenal ulcer may bring the patient face to face with his problems again, and it may be this, not the medication, that causes reactive tension or depression.

Carcinoma of the pancreas

Carcinoma of the pancreas arises in men three times as often as in women, in the age range 50-70. In 10-20 per cent of cases psychiatric symptoms antedate the diagnosis by as long as 12 months. It is important for the psychiatrist to consider this if he is sent an obviously depressed man complaining of abdominal pain. Characteristically the mood is low, with a sense of doom but not of guilt: there is intractable insomnia, poor appetite and marked weight loss. The patient is pale and later develops a lemon tinge from jaundice. Treatment of the depression in its own right may ameliorate the patient's total suffering, in conjunction with specific measures. Trazodone (50-250 mg in 24 hours) or clomipramine (30-150 mg) may help, with the major dose at night. Clomipramine is not available in the US.

Pancreatitis

Pancreatitis is also frequently associated with psychiatric symptoms. These may continue or become obvious for the first time even after an acute episode has subsided. In 53 per cent there is an acute organic brain syndrome including transient hallucinations; in less severe reactions 29 per cent show impairment of memory, 26 per cent inability to concentrate, 23 per cent agitation, 19 per cent confabulation (Schuster, 1980). Treatment is as for other organic brain syndromes (see Chapter 3).

Most but not all patients with chronic pancreatitis are alcoholics. They are often beset by anxiety, depression, insomnia and central abdominal pain, the latter readily leading to narcotic addiction. In this case the physican may want help with the reduction of opiate dosage: neuroleptics such as haloperidol or chlorpromazine will prevent withdrawal symptoms and have inherent calming and analgesic effects. In such cases haloperidol may be given 4 times daily initially, reducing every few days; chlorpromazine may be used similarly with 25-50 mg doses.

Constipation

Constipation, vaguely 'a change in bowel habit', has been well publicised as an early warning of rectal or colonic cancer. Cancer-phobic men, who are likely to be primarily depressive or tensely obsessional, frequently focus on their bowels, whereas similarly phobic women look towards breast or uterus for fatal trouble. Constipation may be due to organic obstruction, neurological disorder, motility problems including diverticular disease and the atony of old age and little exercise. Causes of particular psychiatric concern include nutritional as in anorexia nervosa; inhibition following painful surgery or piles; slow-down as in depression or hypothyroidism; the late result of purgative abuse; chronic organic brain syndromes; and medication including such psychotropics as tricyclic antidepressants,

MAOIs, neuroleptics and anticholinergics.

Purgative abuse

Purgative abuse usually affects women. The younger adults often have frank anorexia or bulimia nervosa, sometimes taking 100 or more senna tablets daily. There is also a group of women of 50-plus who may have anorexia tardive or are merely anxious and obsessional, with an overvalued concept of inner cleanliness. Management involves retraining of the colon, with enemas initially, and is likely to take many months. At worst the colon becomes a drainpipe with no controls. Psychiatric treatment comprises psychotherapeutic support aimed at rebuilding self-esteem, new interests and more effective relationships. Antidepressants may have a secondary place.

Irritable colon

Irritable colon is a common functional disorder of mobility involving high but variable intracolonic pressure. It effects predominantly females, from childhood to over 60 but particularly adolescents and young adults. Characteristics are colicky pain or constant aching especially on the left, the passage of hard pellets and periods of constipation or diarrhoea (Connell, 1973). Gastroenterologists usually try antispasmodics, with variable and often short-lived success, and send the non-responders to psychiatrists. Whatever may be the initial cause, emotional tension makes matters worse. Support and encouragement with the hurdles of becoming an independent adult are needed, including help with expressing emotions. Relaxation therapy followed up by an audiotape must include specifically the organs inside the abdomen and reassurance that the patient is well-liked and safely surrounded by beneficent feelings. Results are usually gratifyingly good, but the patient may return years later for a boost when a new life-change looms.

Aerophagy

Aerophagy often exacerbates the symptoms of irritable colon and of other abdominal disorders, organic or functional. It is natural to swallow excessively in such circumstances as extreme nervousness,

115

as in an interview, or if there is epigastric discomfort for whatever reason. Aerophagy may become habitual in generally anxious or dyspeptic people, or with alcohol drinking. It produces uncomfortable bloating, colic en route and flatulence.

Case: Mrs Z., a timid lady of 65 raised to rigid standards, was shy in company. This led to aerophagy, discomfort and embarrassing flatulence. She became virtually housebound and her medically trained husband exhausted his colleagues with the problem while avoiding all psychiatric consultation. It transpired that the disorder had developed at a time of family humiliation, when their son was sent to prison. She had had to swallow her pride while feeling that everyone around was aware of some badness about her, much as they could detect the smell of flatus emanating from her. Awareness of the habit and supervised practice in avoiding it may be helped by anxiolytic or antidepresssant medication: Mrs Z. was chronically agitated and depressed.

Ulcerative colitis

Ulcerative colitis presents with devastating episodes of bloody diarrhoea, frequently complicated by infection, haemorrhage or sinus formation. It usually develops between the ages of 20 and 40, key years for romantic, reproductive, career and social activities. The organic aetiology is uncertain, but Engel (1974) believes that the disorder is at least precipitated by the threat of disruption of a dependent relationship. Whether emotional factors are an integral part of ulcerative colitis or result from it, patients are often histrionically distressed when physical symptoms are either fulminant or in remission.

Relationships come under strain from the illness. Partners may find the situation unbearable and withdraw: or if they remain closely involved are likely to do so because of their own neurotic needs. Parents — understandably mothers in particular — tend to become overprotective and interfering. Patients respond with resentment, clinging and petulance. Support for the patients and mediation between family members may be needed, with psychotropic medication if depressive, paranoid or anxiety symptoms reach unacceptable levels. The use of corticosteroids may be a factor in psychiatric symptomatology. If major surgery in the form of colectomy and ileostomy is contemplated, explanation, support and reassurance, preferably from an ileostomy counsellor, are required. Colitis sufferers often respond to the challenge with courage and competence: see below.

Regional ileitis: Crohn's disease

This affects both large and small intestine with mucosal ulceration and narrowing of the lumen. Again, young adults are frequently affected: symptoms are similar to those in ulcerative colitis with more continuous pain and episodes of severe colic and other indications of obstruction. Electrolyte disturbances and anaemia are common, and psychological disturbance may be precipitated also by corticosteroids. Since surgical resection is often disappointing because of the patchy development of the disease, these patients are likely to have years of ill-health, strain and insecurity, and most will require psychiatric support at some stage for affective disturbance. Patients are likely to be depressed, even suicidal, and anxiously obsessional. Dependency, preoccupation with the bowels and social withdrawal are understandable reactions to the disease. Of course emotional upsets make matters worse but are neither necessary nor sufficient in the causation of the illness. Often a psychiatric opinion is requested when the patient's complaints and demands for analgesia outstrip what the physician regards as appropriate.

The time-lag between, for instance, restoration of electrolyte balance and secure affective functioning must be recognised. On the other hand opiate analgesia is in itself pleasant and may be asked for too freely (see Chapter 4). Tact is required to satisfy both physician and patient while introducing a relaxing antidepressant such as trimipramine or maprotiline, each with 25 mg doses, or trazodone, 50 mg two to four times daily, to take the edge off the patient's distress and to enable some reduction in analgesia. The patient will be angry if she feels discounted as 'psychiatric' and that she is being 'fobbed off with tranquillisers'. Consistency between all staff in what the patient is told is vital.

Post-hepatitis depression

Infective hepatitis, in common with some other viral illnesses such as influenza and infectious mononucleosis, is frequently followed for up to three months by fatigue, poor appetite, low mood and lack of interest. This form of reactive depression responds to antidepressant treatment with, for instance maprotiline or clomipramine: either at a dosage of 75-150 mg in 24 hours. (Clomipramine is not available in the US.)

Hepatic encephalopathy

Hepatic encephalopathy affects mainly (70 per cent) alcoholics. It is associated with liver cell failure and, in cirrhosis, the shunting of portal venous blood directly into the systemic circulation without detoxification. Nitrogen products in particular are damaging. Metabolic failure from progressive hepatic disease leads insidiously into a chronic organic brain syndrome with increasing episodes of disorientation, delirium and finally coma. The early stages amount to no more than exaggeration of existing personality traits with sweeps of depression and daytime hypersomnia. Even at this stage the electroencephalogram shows slowing.

Difficulties in concentration and lack of intellectual initiative and interest follow, and are accompanied, significantly, by constructional dyspraxia: shown by deterioration in handwriting and difficulty in copying a shape. Next, episodes of disorientation, especially spatial, leading to getting lost, arise, as does inappropriate behaviour, including violence. Increasing confusion and drowsiness or frank delirium usher in hepatic coma, which may continue, fluctuant, for many weeks. Ascites and jaundice are common. At this stage the characteristic flapping tremor, asterixis, may appear, and such signs as hyperreflexia, cogwheeling and extensor plantar responses.

The stigmata of chronic alcoholism are likely to be present but may lead a false diagnostic trail. Hepatic encephalopathy may be mistaken for delirium tremens or for alcoholic depression. The differentiation is important since the sedating medication used in DTs, or an antidepressant, may tip the patient into unconsciousness when drug metabolism in the liver is in abeyance. The giving of a protein load which worsens the symptoms in hepatic encephalopathy has been suggested as a diagnostic test, but is dangerous. In the EEG, alpha rhythms are likely to be replaced by bilaterally synchronous delta waves (Victor, 1983). Treatment is urgently medical: emptying the bowel, restricting protein intake, and the use of neomycin or lactulose, and frusemide if necessary. Psychiatric management may be a necessary adjunct if the patient is disturbed or needs preparation and support for transplant. Droperidol and haloperidol are short-acting, do not depend on hepatic detoxification and may be given by any route.

Nutritional encephalopathies are usually also alcohol-related in the Western world (see below and also Chapter 15).

Postoperative syndromes

Postgastrectomy syndrome

In some patients an exaggeration of the normal physiological response to food occurs, with palpitations, flushing, sweating and drowsiness either immediately after food or an hour later. This is the 'dumping syndrome' and appears to be related to undue reactive hypoglycaemia (Chapter 9). This syndrome usually improves with dietary emphasis away from rapidly absorbable carbohydrates, physiological readjustment over time, and if necessary medication such as anticholinergics to slow down gastric emptying. Dumping is not a key factor in the postgastrectomy syndrome which affects up to 50 per cent of patients. It comprises excessive fatigue and muscular weakness, sometimes accompanied by frank anxiety or depression, and interferes with the patients' normal activities. One-third accept lower-powered lower-paid employment than previously.

Those in whom the syndrome persists for months or more and also includes pain are more likely to have undergone surgery for intractable pain than for acute, incontrovertible pathology. Among the latter group immediate postoperative progress is most favourable in patients who are moderately anxious beforehand and were informed rather than reassured about the likely outcome (Morgan, 1973). In the persistent preoperative pain group, postoperative prognosis is better if there is adequate environmental support, i.e. job, income, home, marriage and a secure childhood experience. A high neuroticism score on the Eysenck Personality Inventory preoperatively indicates a predisposition to respond maladaptively to stress, and is predictive of an unsatisfactory outcome in these cases (Drinkwater and McColl, 1976). After selective vagotomy for peptic ulcer there is a 21 per cent failure rate: one-third have recurrent ulceration; one-third develop a postgastrectomy syndrome as disabling as their original condition; and the remainder have ongoing neurotic problems (Alexander-Williams *et al.*, 1977). Depression, anxiety or hysterical benefit may maintain the patient's symptoms in the absence of continuing organic pathology. Pain may also have become a conditioned response if it has been associated with other stimuli, sensory or emotional: these alone may then act as triggers to the familiar pain. It is unfortunate if the work environment becomes such a trigger.

Although preoperative predictive assessment is ideal, it is usually

119

after surgery, if recovery lags, that a psychiatric opinion is invited. Any of the range of psychiatric conditions just mentioned, and of course concealed alcohol use, may be a major factor in the patient's symptoms. His pride needs to be considered sympathetically if psychotropic medication and serial discussions with a psychiatrist are envisaged.

Late effects of partial gastrectomy may be those of *hydroxocobalamin deficiency*: depression, paranoid states, with or without megaloblastic anaemia, glossitis, weakness, paraesthesiae, and subacute combined degeneration of the cord. Cerebral damage may become permanent so psychiatric symptoms demand prompt treatment. Diagnosis of vitamin B_{12} deficiency is made specifically by the Schilling test; low serum B_{12} is a useful screen. Treatment is with parenteral hydroxocabalamin, but psychotropics may be needed temporarily and occasionally long-term cyanocobalamin is recommended instead of hydroxocobalamin in the US.

Postcholecystectomy syndrome

A more or less unsatisfactory outcome occurs in 40 per cent of patients; 10 per cent have dyspepsia; 24 per cent mild pain; and 3 per cent severe pain. As with gastric surgery the patients who respond least well have had vague symptoms rather than typical recurrent biliary colic, with stones. Bloating, heartburn, flatulence and right upper quadrant pain after meals may result from functionally disordered gastrointestinal motility. This may be made worse postoperatively by elevated cholecystokinin levels. Psychological factors and treatment are similar to those in irritable colon: see above. Many patients continue with faulty dietary habits and remain oveweight, but are indignant if such sensitive subjects are raised.

Adjustment to ostomy surgery

Ileostomy and colostomy each impose a new method of waste disposal; external deformity; and the attachment of prosthetic appliances. They induce anxieties about smell, leakage, and acceptability to others socially and especially sexually. On the whole patients fare better psychologically after ileostomy than colostomy, largely because of the nature of the underlying disease. Colectomy with permanent ileostomy is usually considered worthwhile compared with their preoperative condition by patients with ulcerative colitis. Nevertheless at least half of them experience discomfort and unease with their ileostomy, and anxiety about the attitude of key others. Colostomy for large bowel cancer, by contrast, is accompanied by feelings of depression, shame, helplessness, anger, worthlessness — and isolation. Unlike ileostomy patients who cannot expect to control their outflow, colostomy patients are encouraged to learn to regulate their bowel actions. Failure is humiliating and may resurrect unhappy memories of early training.

Preoperative assessment and preparation have a major influence on postoperative adjustment. Patients with ulcerative colitis who have suffered for only a few months, however acutely, adjust less well than longer-term sufferers. Prophylactic surgery in symptomless familial multiple polyposis is also difficult to accept. Preoperative counselling should include the patient's spouse and other family members.

Immediate postoperative response to ostomy includes revulsion and helplessness. Either denial or regression may serve a useful temporary purpose in getting the patient through the first impact without unbearable anxiety and depression. Regression may reveal itself in constant demands and complaints, with no attempt to learn self-care; nursing and medical staff need to be prepared to put up with this attitude for the initial period. Longer-term adjustment depends on the patient's inherent strengths and support from professionals, counsellor, and, importantly, family, friends and work colleagues. Self-help groups help those who are naturally 'clubbable'.

Sexual maladjustment may result from the patient's loss of libido from depression, or debility from the disease; impotence from accidental damage to the sympathetic nerves usually from pelvic dissection in rectal carcinoma; feelings of anxiety; or a negative reaction by the partner. In contrast to gastrectomy patients, 90 per cent of ostomy patients continue in the same jobs. Marital tension is attributed to the stoma in 10 per cent of marriages and in 2 per cent the marriage crumbles (Burnham *et al.*, 1977). It is those who are not established in marriage who suffer most in their relations.

Case: Miss N.A., 34, had an unhappy upbringing as the only child and go-between of parents who did not speak to each other for months at a time. She escaped gratefully into nursing where she did well until her ulcerative colitis developed. Her current boyfriend broke off the relationship and a similar break-up occurred after her ileostomy later. Depression and loneliness manifested in pain; in an effort to remain at work N.A. abused both alcohol and pethidine. Jobless, her suicidal depression is understandable.

Ongoing support and encouragement during a restructuring of social life and expectations is needed, with specific psychotropic therapy during episodes of clinical depression, tension or paranoia.

Nutritional deficiency syndromes

In Western culture the commonest cause of nutritional deficiency is alcohol abuse. Alcohol excess is associated with disorders in every bodily system, but essentially and most intimately the gastrointestinal apparatus. The transient inflammatory response of the oesophageal mucosa as a draught of brandy or slivovitz descends is appreciated as a warm glow. Similar damage affects the lower reaches of the tract but does not impinge upon subjective awareness. Acute or chronic gastritis, duodenitis, pancreatitis and hepatitis with finally cirrhosis and occasionally hepatic carcinoma, and also colonic disorders, may all be due to alcohol.

Nutritional deficiencies associated with alcoholism include generalised malnutrition and specific vitamin deficiencies. Alcohol, nicotine and illegal social drugs with the exception of cannabis all reduce appetite. Since alcohol provides calories, albeit of limited usefulness and a spurious feeling of warmth from peripheral vasodilatation, it is particularly likely to lead to relative starvation.

Others at risk of malnutrition are the elderly, the mentally impaired, and inmates of institutions which are inadequately funded. Simple undernourishment leads to weight loss and irritability, intolerance to noise, restlessness, hypochondriasis, and an uncharacteristic callousness and lack of concern for others. Obsessionality is common, and is notable in patients with anorexia nervosa and in deprived prisoners of war.

Symptoms of vitamin lack usually occur when an acute demand arises in circumstances of chronic deficiency.

Thiamine (B_1) deficiency

Thiamine is derived mainly from expensive fish and meat foods and is essential for the utilisation of carbohydrates. The brain is unusually vulnerable to disturbance in carbohydrate metabolism and thus to thiamine deficiency since glucose is its sole source of energy and it runs at a high metabolic rate. Heavy alcohol consumption without solid food, prolonged gastrointestinal upset impairing absorption, gastric carcinoma or surgery, and strict vegetarianism may lead to thiamine deficiency. Early symptoms may go unrecognised; they comprise weakness, irritability, forgetfulness, insomnia and apathy. With acute deficiency, made worse if a carbohydrate load is given for instance in starvation or alcohol excess, Wernicke's encephalopathy may suddenly and disastrously develop. Korsakov's syndrome is a common sequel. Constitutional transketolase deficiency may be an additional adverse factor in alcoholics. Alcoholic vagrants, because of their poor diet, are at particular risk and should routinely receive parenteral vitamins B and C if they present in casualty or the emergency room (see Chapter 5).

Nicotinic acid deficiency

Again the poor, the elderly, the institutionalised and those who have had gastrointestinal surgery or ongoing disease are likely to suffer. Alcoholics, especially those who drink beer, which contains nicotinic acid, are less liable to suffer from deficiency of this vitamin than of B_1 or B_{12}. Early symptoms are neurasthenic, but a subacute or acute brain syndrome, and occasionally stupor, may suddenly appear. The tongue may be red and sore but neurological signs indicate a multivitamin deficiency. Dramatic improvement occurs within 24 hours of oral or intramuscular nicotinamide.

Hydroxocobalamin (B_{12}) deficiency

This occurs with impaired absorption after partial gastrectomy or intestinal resection, visceral malignancy, strict veganism, chronic diarrhoea and intestinal parasitism. It is considered above in relation to gastrectomy.

Folic acid deficiency

This may result from prolonged phenytoin administration in epilepsy, and also arises in the elderly and ill-nourished, including alcoholics. The effects resemble B_{12} deficiency with megaloblastic anaemia, glossitis, anorexia and diarrhoea. Depression and dementia may at least be aggravated by folate lack (Crammer, 1983). Red cell rather than serum folate levels should be estimated and in case of deficiency folic acid tablets, 5 mg twice daily, may be given.

Pyridoxine (B_6) deficiency

The need for pyridoxine is increased by a high intake of animal protein, treatment with oestrogens including the contraceptive pill, hydrazides and MAOIs. Patients developing a peripheral neuropathy on an MAOI should be given pyridoxine 50 mg b.d. The rationale for giving pyridoxine for premenstrual tension is tenuous, but in constitutionally susceptible people an organic brain syndrome may occur, especially in alcoholics, from pyridoxine deficiency. The dosage should then be 200 mg daily.

123

Pyrodixone should not be given to parkinsonian patients under treatment with levodopa since it enhances the action of peripheral decarboxylase. It may do no harm if a decarboxylase inhibitor is included.

REFERENCES

Ackerman, S.H. and Weiner, H. (1976) 'Peptic Ulcer Disease: Some Considerations for Psychosomatic Research', in Hill, O.W. (Ed.) *Modern Trends in Psychosomatic Medicine — 3*, Butterworths, London

Alexander-Williams, J., Betts, T.A. and Pidd, S. (1977) 'Psychiatric Disturbance and the Effects of Gastric Operations', *Clinics in Gastroenterology, 6*, 694-8

Burnham, W.R., Leonard-Jones, J.E. and Brooke, E.N. (1977) 'Sexual Problems among Married Ileostomates', *Gut, 18*, 673-7

Connell, A.M. (1973) (1973) 'Functional Aspects of Colonic Motility: Constipation', in Lindmer, A.E. (Ed.) *Emotional Factors in Gastrointestinal Illness*, Excerpta Medica, Amsterdam

Crammer, J.L. (1983) 'Nutritional Abnormalities', in Lader, M.H. (Ed.) *Mental Disorders and Somatic Illness*, Cambridge University Press, Cambridge

Drinkwater, J.E. and McColl, I. (1976) Chapter 15, in Howells, J.G. (Ed.) *Modern Perspectives in the Psychiatric Aspects of Surgery*, Macmillan, London

Engel, G.L. (1974) 'Psychological Aspects of Gastrointestinal Disorders', in Ariete, S. and Reiser, M.F. (Eds) *American Handbook of Psychiatry — 2*, Basic Books, New York

Gomez, J. (1984) 'Abdominal Pain', *Update, 1*, 61-6

Gomez, J. and Dally, P. (1977) 'Psychologically Mediated Abdominal Pain in Surgical and Medical Outpatient Clinics', *British Medical Journal, 1*, 1451-3

Mirsky, I.A. (1958) 'Physiological, Psychologic, and Social Determinants in the Etiology of Duodenal Ulcer', *American Journal of Digestive Disease, 3*, 285-314

Morgan, D. (1973) 'Psychosomatic Aspects of Peptic Ulcer Disease', in Munro, A. (Ed.) *Psychosomatic Medicine*, Churchill-Livingstone, Edinburgh and New York

Nichol, A.R. (1982) 'Psychogenic Abdominal Pain in Childhood', *British Journal of Hospital Medicine, 27*, 351-3

Schuster, M.M. (1980) 'Psychiatric Manifestations of Gastrointestinal Disorders', in Hall, R.C.W. (Ed.) Psychiatric Presentations of Medical Illnesses, Spectrum, New York

Victor, M. (1983) 'Mental Disorders Due to Alcoholism', in Lader, M.H. (Ed.) *Mental Disorders and Somatic Illness*, Cambridge University Press, Cambridge

Wangensteen, S.L. and Golden, G.T. (1973) 'Acute "Stress" Ulcers of the Stomach: a Review', *American Surgery, 39*, 562-7

8

Liaison in Obstetrics and Gynaecology

Nowhere is psychiatric liaison needed more than in this field. Puberty for the female is marked by dramatic, even alarming menarche. The flow of blood conveys lack of control, and warns of the perils of childbirth, which is now a possibility. No wonder that some inhibited middle-class girls, perhaps grappling with school or college examinations, attempt to reject these female aspects of growing up and develop anorexia nervosa (see Chapter 9).

DYSMENORRHOEA

Dysmenorrhoea, the uterine equivalent of irritable colon, affects a large proportion of girls, particularly on the first day of the period, and is sometimes severe enough to prevent their going to school or engaging in some other activity. Dysmenorrhoea does not usually arise until the menses become ovular, up to five years after menarche. It may continue for a few months only, persist until parity, or rarely continue indefinitely. *Mittelschmerz*, occurring at the time of ovulation, is a minor pain, more likely in those complaining of period pain.

Dysmenorrhoea may interrupt studies or interfere with normal social and occupational functioning for much of the month. For those of immature personality, periods pose a long-acting threat of maternity, meaning responsibility and identification with mother. Meanwhile dysmenorrhoea provides an avoidance mechanismn for any disliked activity, a source of sympathy and perhaps such tangible rewards as analgesia or alcohol. It is generally accepted that often the patients who suffer most are those whose mothers gave a negative view of sex and men, and provide a model of female martyrdom. Dysmenorrhoea is made worse by anxiety, tension states, and reactive depression; it may be involved in hysterical mechanisms. It has a positive association with menstrual irregularity and the premenstrual syndrome later.

A few months on the oral contraceptive pill will settle the symptom, at least temporarily, but this does not unravel the conflicts and uncertainties surrounding it, nor reduce the likelihood of further gynaecologically attributed problems. Realistic discussion of facts and feelings in a finite number of four to six sessions should be offered. If there is much anxiety, diazepam, with its mental and muscle-relaxing properties, should be given for three days per cycle starting on the day before the period: 2-5 mg twice a day should be adequate. In those whose life is disrupted by dysmenorrhoea, even on the pill, and in whom symptoms of tension and depression can be elicited, a course of phenelzine (MAOI) or trazodone will be needed for psychotherapy to be effective. Penelzine should be given in daily dosage of 15-60 mg, all before 4 pm; trazodone in the range 50-250 mg in the 24 hours.

MENSTRUAL IRREGULARITIES

Menstrual irregularities encompass anything from undue frequency to absence, length more than seven days, heavy flow, or hardly noticeable bleeding. They usually occur in the context of emotional disturbance: the strain of being a student away from home for the first time, guilt or anxiety over sexual activity, dietary and other chaos in bulimia nervosa, or the onset of a functional psychosis. Except in the latter case, requiring treatment in its own right, therapy is similar to that in dysmenorrhoea. An important group are those with unsatisfactory marriages, anxious to avoid pregnancy, whose marital lives revolve round their menstrual status. Menstrual irregularities, in the absence of clear gynaecological pathology, are used as a reason to press for early hysterectomy. Those patients accustomed to using their symptoms, however innocently, to manipulate are likely to develop abdominal pain and other symptoms some weeks postoperatively and bemoan their inability to conceive. A course of couples therapy to improve communication and understanding in the marriage is essential before surgery is considered.

THE PREMENSTRUAL SYNDROME

Every psychiatrist can expect referrals from the gynaecologists of difficult women often in their thirties said to be suffering from the premenstrual syndrome but unresponsive to the usual ploys of progesterone or an oral contraceptive. Physicians of the Hippocratic school were familiar with the psychosomatic discomforts of the premenstruum, and those of the nineteenth century were still concerned with women's 'periodical ordeal' (Clare, 1982, 1983). It was not until 1953, however, that Dalton and Greene gave the premenstrual syndrome (PMS) its name, and in the 1980s it gained headline status as an acceptable plea of mitigation in the British Courts for three serious crimes: arson, assault and manslaughter (Dalton, 1982). Controversy continues unabated over its symptomatology, aetiology and treatment (Jones, 1983).

Significant associations with PMS include neurotic psychiatric morbidity, as assessed by the General Health Questionnaire and clinically (Clare, 1983). Most women with neurotic disorders also complain of PMS, and the psychological components are particularly severe compared with those with PMS but no psychiatric disorder. Marital dysfunction, whether or not there is psychiatric symptomatology, is almost invariable. Fifty per cent of PMS patients have dysmenorrhoea, and many have long-lasting or irregular periods. Neuroticism scores on the Eysenck Personality Inventory are raised in PMS and menstrual irregularity but not with dysmenorrhoea on its own. Somewhat unexpectedly there is no statistically significant association between PMS and impaired general social adjustment, parity or taking the oral contraceptive pill.

A fatal outcome from accident, suicide or illness is found more frequently in the second part of the menstrual cycle. Studies involving crime and non-fatal deliberate self-harm are retrospective and scientifically unsatisfactory so far.

Symptomatology

According to Dalton this covers a broad range, including asthmatic and epileptic fits if they occur cyclically in the luteal phase, with a symptom-free phase of at least seven days post-menstrually. A diagnostic aid is a chart on which the patient records her symptoms and her periods. Generally recognised manifestations of PMS come in three groups:

Physical: weight gain, bloated feeling, tender breasts, abdominal pain, backache, headache; nausea; stiffness
Behavioural: clumsiness; increased proneness to accidents; decreased

normal activity; reduced efficiency; aggressive responses
Psychological: tearfulness, tension, irritability, initial insomnia, impaired concentration, moodiness, a sense of loneliness.

Aetiology

A physiological substrate to PMS seems obvious but careful studies have failed to find the expected flattening of the progesterone curve in the luteal phase except in one-third of cases, nor is there an increased prolactin level. The interesting claim by some women, and put forward by Backstrom *et al.* (1981), of continuing PMS after hysterectomy has been shown to be largely subjective and unrelated to hormonal status (Slade, 1984). It may be that PMS comprises a cluster of disparate conditions of varying aetiology (Van Keep and Lehert, 1981), or that aberrant endorphin release is involved (Reid and Yen, 1981), but it is certain that there is a large psychological element and sexual disturbance, probably mediated through the hypothalamo-pituitary-gonadal axis. Excess of prolactin is one of the more recent suggestions in the aetiology of PMS (Donovan, 1985).

Management

An 88 per cent placebo response makes the assessment of treatment difficult, particularly in a disorder that only presents for part of each month (Mattsson and Schoultz, 1974). Rational treatments tried but not established as better than placebo include:

1. progesterone, aiming to increase an unproven low level;
2. bromocriptine, to reduce an unproven high level of prolactin;
3. pyridoxine, to correct an unproven functional deficiency;
4. spironolactone, to counteract unproven changes in aldosterone level;
5. diuretics, to reduce supposed water retention.

Psychoactive drugs, including lithium, anxiolytics and antidepressants, have not been found to have a significant therapeutic effect when tested under strict conditions.

Recommendation

A condition that affects 95 per cent of menstruating women enough for them to be aware of it, and causes 40 per cent sufficient distress to ask for medical help, cannot be ignored. Individual psychotherapy aimed at enhancing self-esteem and reducing tension, and couples therapy to create greater sexual harmony, should be used in addition to whichever chemical therapy suits the patient best. The dignity of receiving medication, and the active or placebo effect will reinforce psychological treatment.

PELVIC PAIN ATTRIBUTED TO GYNAECOLOGICAL DISEASE

Lower abdominal pain has different connotations among the young and sexually active and among older women. The former worry about infection or pregnancy, the latter about cancer. When pelvic inflammatory disease (PID) arises in the psychologically immature, it is sometimes associated with tension and guilt, anxiety about possible sterility later, or worries concerning current sexual activity and its risks. An episode of PID, adequately treated, frequently initiates a girl of hysterical personality into a long career of abdominal pain with or without physical disease. Pelvic pain due neither to PID or endometriosis nor other gynaecological pathology is often associated with chronic tension or depression, made understandable from a carefully elicited history.

Case 1: A 23-year-old nun, regretting what she had renounced as a woman, had crippling abdominal pain which subsided when she was released from her order.

Case 2: A 50-year-old woman married late and her husband died of myocardial infarction on their honeymoon. She apparently coped well and returned to work, but within a few months developed aching pelvic pain (worse in the mornings), and loss of energy, sleep and appetite. Her bereavement depression responded well to amitriptyline.

Post-termination mourning may also reflect in pelvic pain, and the nulliparous woman of 40-plus may suffer abdominal aching. Such cases are a form of reactive depression and may respond to doxepin, maprotiline, mianserin and flupenthixol together, or an MAOI; and discussion.

129

POST-HYSTERECTOMY DEPRESSION

Depression following hysterectomy is relatively common, occurring in more than 7 per cent of cases, significantly more than in a comparable group of women undergoing cholecystectomy (Barker, 1968). Pelvic operations in general, including prostatectomy in men, are more often associated with depressive reactions than surgery elsewhere: perhaps because of sexual connotations and damage to self-esteem. Gynaecologists sometimes ask for an assessment of the likelihood of depression in a particular case. A previous episode of affective illness increases the risk tenfold, and those without significant gynaecological pathology are more susceptible to depression than patients who have a pelvic tumour, benign or malignant. Oopherectomy does not increase the risk however, so hormonal effects are unlikely to be highly relevant. A postoperative confusional state does not make later affective disturbance any more likely (Whitlock, 1982). The depression is unlikely to arise within the first few postoperative weeks; the timescale is such that the gynaecologist is taken by surprise when his 'successful' case develops depression. Turpin and Heath (1979) describe a time lag of six months to two years, much as may occur with a bereavement. Psychological and social factors are obviously important and, as with mastectomy, the attitude of the husband is of paramount importance (Gath and Rose, 1985).

In patients considered to be vulnerable, a pre- and postoperative exploration of feelings with the woman, and her husband also on at least one occasion, may have a prophylactic effect. Since plasma tryptophan levels are depleted in conjunction with the post-hysterectomy drop in oestrogen levels, a reasonable manoeuvre, with no risk of side-effects, is the administration of L-tryptophan, 500-1000 mg at night for a few months. Tryptophan is the precursor of the neurotransmitter, serotonin.

PREGNANCY

Whether planned, unplanned or unwanted, pregnancy is only uncommonly associated with the onset of psychiatric illness severe enough to require admission, although minor emotional disturbances are common enough. Marcé, in the mid-nineteenth century (1858), noticed that pregnancy can alter a woman's state of mind in opposite directions: some become calmer, others more anxious. This difference is likely to have been a function of the stage of pregnancy.

First trimester

The characteristic feelings are anxiety and ambivalence. Because of the latter, miscarriage is less upsetting than later. A woman who has previously had a termination of pregnancy, legal or illegal, is more vulnerable to neurotic anxiety-depression at this stage; earlier spontaneous miscarriage does not have this association (Kumar and Robson, 1978).

Second trimester

The mood is stable and self-confident, with an increase of drive. Anxiety and ambivalence subside, as does depression if present earlier. Miscarriage at this stage is upsetting, but termination does not usually have psychiatric sequelae, although foetal movements may have been felt (Brewer, 1978).

Third trimester

Understandably, lethargy takes over. In the last few weeks fears about labour and about whether the baby will be perfect may develop. The greatest reassurance derives from getting to know the midwife, obstetrician and ward sister at the hospital, or their equivalent with a domiciliary delivery.

Minor disturbances in pregnancy include mood swings, variations in energy, and unaccustomed dietary cravings and aversions for which there seems no rational cause. Nausea and vomiting are commonplace in the early weeks but vanish like snow in the sun during the second trimester. Occasionally, vomiting becomes severe and does not remit (hyperemesis gravidarum). Although obstetric factors are accountable in some cases, others are largely psychogenic and occur usually in women of immature, hysterical personality feeling insecure perhaps because of an inadequate, culturally different or much older husband. Hyperemesis is dangerous to both mother and foetus and requires treatment with a sedating phenothiazine such as chlorpromazine, relaxation and supportive psychotherapy.

Patients with neuroses need particular care during pregnancy. Like those mentally impaired they tend to have curtailed periods of gestation, more complications during delivery, and babies with lower birth weights than others. The support and observation these patients require should not be backed up by medication, except in those either with hysterical personality disorders or impaired intellectually, who may deliberately cause vaginal bleeding. Admission, observation, relaxation, support and chlorpromazine are required for these.

Psychoses are not precipitated by pregnancy alone, and those patients with established schizophrenic or manic-depressive illness are not likely to relapse before the baby is born.

Psychotropic medication during pregnancy

Schizophrenics on neuroleptics should continue their drug regimen during pregnancy and after labour. Relapse is likely with reduction of the dosage, and there appears to be no risk to the foetus in continuing. The amount of, for instance, chlorpromazine getting into breast milk is minute, so breast-feeding does not militate against neuroleptic use (Brockington and Kumar, 1982; Oppenheim, 1985).

In the case of manic-depressive patients established on lithium, the situation is different. There is some evidence of teratogenicity with lithium, and theoretically impairment of foetal thyroid function might be expected. The time of delivery is particularly dangerous for a woman on lithium since the plasma level may suddenly treble. Lithium also comes through into breast milk, at less than half the serum level. However, an attack of diarrhoea or other upset in mother or infant may cause a sharp rise in lithium concentration, with undesirable effects. Patients on lithium should use contraceptives until they plan to conceive, when they should stop the medication. Relapse is unusual in pregnancy but common puerperally; the mother should be guided towards bottle-feeding and restart her lithium after delivery. Dosage is monitored to maintain a serum level of 0.6-0.9 mmol/(mEq/l).

Psychotropic medication has been viewed askance in pregnancy since the thalidomide tragedy, and women who may become pregnant should not be prescribed medication for the milder neurotic disorders. Since women have conceived while on almost every psychotropic medication without a significant increase in abnormal babies, the risks are clearly small; however, although MAOIs appear to have no teratogenetic effect, they must be withheld shortly before labour because of their interaction with narcotic analgesics. Tricyclic and related antidepressants may very slightly increase the risk of foetal maldevelopment, and are excreted in the milk at a low level. Benzodiazepines such as diazepam and chlordiazepoxide may lead to oral cleft defects if used in early pregnancy. When given later, for treatment of pre-eclamptic toxaemia, benzodiazepines may induce hypotonia in the infant, or withdrawal symptoms. Barbiturates should be avoided in pregnancy but this may not be practicable in epilepsy.

The risk of malformation is 6.6 per cent compared with 2.7 per cent for controls, but may be due to the epilepsy as much as the antiepileptic drugs.

Electroconvulsive therapy

Severe depression is rare in pregnancy but when it occurs ECT is not contraindicated. The muscle relaxant succinyl choline does not pass into the foetal circulation, and the uterus is not involved in the muscular contractions of the fit. Nevertheless, external foetal monitoring and obstetric liaison are needed with ECT in pregnancy.

Alcohol (see Chapter 15)

The foetal alcohol syndrome was described by the ancients and rediscovered 20 years ago (Lemoine *et al.*, 1968). Binge drinking in particular, in the first trimester, is likely to cause facial, head and cardiac malformations; in the second trimester short stature and psychomotor disturbance, and in the third trimester low birth weight. A low IQ is general. Although it is desirable to persuade a mother to give up alcohol when she is pregnant or lactating, disulfiram must not be used: it is associated with limb deformities.

Tobacco

Smoking and drinking often go together. Both nicotine and carbon monoxide are potentially harmful to the foetus. Low birth weight is associated with smoking in the second half of pregnancy: each cigarette daily is calculated to reduce the baby's weight by 8 g and to increase the risk of perinatal mortality. Problems with school work are likelier, in such children. Efforts to persuade pregnant patients to give up smoking are worthwhile.

Illegal social drugs

Regular narcotic use results in reduced fertility, but pregnant girls with multiple social problems are sometimes also on heroin. They may look ill and undernourished, and show needle tracks on their arms and hands: often they deny involvement with drugs for fear of sanctions.

Complications include infection from injection sites, including abscesses and hepatitis B. Heroin is not teratogenic but may cause growth impairment, foetal death and withdrawal syndromes in the neonate. Unless the patient agrees to careful detoxification early in pregnancy, the best ploy is to maintain her on oral methadone, including during labour. The baby best responds to 0.1-0.2 mg paregoric six-hourly for a few days; chlorpromazine at a dosage of 2.2 mg/kg/day may be needed for several weeks. Ex-heroin-addict mothers need support, but usually care for their babies adequately. Sudden infant death is more likely than usual if the mother is an ongoing narcotic user. Dipipanone, sometimes marketed with the antiemetic cyclizine, is more likely to be associated with foetal abnormalities than heroin, but has not been regarded as dangerous until recently.

Amphetamines and cocaine are probably teratogens, affecting urogenital and cardiovascular systems, mouth and limbs. Lysergic acid diethylamide may theoretically cause genetic defects, and so may cannabis, but this has not been demonstrated conclusively. None of the stimulant and hallucinogenic drugs produces physical withdrawal symptoms of serious import.

LABOUR

There is hardly time for psychiatric involvement during labour, and frequently the 'highly strung', nervous woman has an easy time, whereas the sensible, controlled type finds it more difficult. This is one of the few situations in which free expression is not only allowed but encouraged. The presence of the father is comforting. Although it is emotionally and physically stressful, acute breakdown in labour is very rare.

> *Case*: A well-known schizophrenic patient, during the third stage, suddenly declared that she had decided against having the baby and was going on a bus. Since she would stay neither on a bed nor on a mattress, she was sedated with intravenous chlorpromazine and the baby was delivered undamaged.

AFTER-BABY BLUES

Eighty per cent of mothers have a period of tearfulness and mild misery starting on the third postnatal day and lasting a few days. Paykel *et al.* (1980) view this as due to the sudden drop in oestrogen and progesterone levels, increasing monoamine oxidase activity with consequent depletion of neurotransmitters, and a sharp rise in prolaction. In Pitt's series (1973) he found that 10.8 per cent of women with blues remained distressed two weeks later. They showed impaired concentration and memory; these he felt were organic in origin, stemming from the hormonal upheaval in particularly susceptible women.

Antenatal fears are associated with increased postnatal unhappiness (Areskog *et al.*, 1984). Peace, privacy and security are necessary for a new mother to regain her emotional balance and begin to form a close, warm two-way relationship with her baby. They are difficult to arrange in the hustle of a hospital (Stein, 1982; Pitt, 1985).

POSTNATAL NEUROSES

These may run on from the blues or arise up to 12 months later. They consist of low mood, anxiety and insomnia. The patient fusses over the baby but has little patience and is only too ready for someone else to look after him. She blames the child for her unhappy state. The father tends to react by being over-solicitous, and the patient's mother by taking over and leaving the patient with no rôle (Baker, 1967). Insight is easily obtained, and the whole family needs support and emotional as well as practical guidance, with the patient and her baby at the centre, the others providing the supporting cast. Sedation for one night's good sleep with, for instance, lorazepam makes a reasonable first start. Antidepressants are contraindicated during breast-feeding but may become necessary, particularly if the depression comes on several months postnatally. Dothiepin, doxepin, maprotiline or lofepramine are suitable (Kumar, 1982). Dothiepin, doxepin and maprotiline may each be given in doses of 75-200 mg daily, either divided or substantially at night. Lofepramine is given in 70 mg doses, two to five times daily as above. However, in the US neither dothiepin nor lofepramine is yet available.

Difficulty in returning to normal sexual activity is mainly a neurotic symptom, but is slightly likelier to be prolonged in a mother who breast-feeds (Alder *et al.*, 1986).

POSTPARTUM PSYCHOSES

Acute organic psychoses are rare these days since puerperfal infections are no longer a problem. Puerperal psychosis is not recognised as an entity in the Ninth Revision of the International Classification of Diseases 1978. Kumar (1983), among others, believes this to be a mistake. What is abundantly clear is that childbirth is a major life event with far-reaching effects. It involves a change of rôle and status for the mother, disruption of her day-to-day activities, a new preoccupying relationship with the baby and a shift in emphasis in relationships already established: all deeply imbued with primitive emotions and meanings. There are also physical, including hormonal, factors. It is unsurprising that the range of functional psychoses as well as reactive neurotic disorders may be precipitated in the susceptible by such an important happening. Functional psychoses arise in one to two per 1000 births, and comprise a large majority of depressive psychoses and a minority of schizophrenic or manic cases. They may come on two days after delivery with a cluster of episodes starting in the first two weeks and again 9-12 months later, making a simple hormonal effect less plausible than in third-day blues, but cortisol adjustments may be involved (Sandler, 1978).

Postpartum depression

A past history of affective illness, and in particular of postnatal depression, makes post-partum depression more likely. The patient often gives an impression of being out of touch, but otherwise the symptoms accord with those of other psychotic depressions: guilt, despair, suicidal ideation and in some cases the idea that the baby should be put away for his own benefit, delusions of persecution and of contaminating others, together with vegetative symptoms.

Treatment is urgent

The patient and baby should be nursed together to prevent his later rejection, but with constant nursing observation. Electroconvulsive therapy and/or tricyclic antidepressant therapy and an antipsychotic tranquilliser are required. The prognosis is good for this episode if the marriage is sound, but the risk of a similar postnatal illness is one in five, increasing sharply with a second episode.

Postnatal schizophrenia

A first episode or a relapse of schizophrenia may be precipitated by the major non-contingent life event of giving birth. Fifteen per cent of these patients have a family history of schizophrenia. The illness comes on suddenly a few days or several months postnatally without warning. Typically the patient develops delusions about the staff and the baby: the latter may be neglected but is seldom harmed. Nevertheless, treatment must include close observation, while keeping patient and baby together, and neuroleptic treatment, establishing the patient on depot injections before discharge. Schizophrenic mothers need support indefinitely, and in the bleak situation of illegitimacy are rarely able to manage to live and look after a child.

Postpartum mania

This is much less common than depression, even in patients with manic-depressive illness, and may be dangerous for the baby but not by any intentional harm. A woman of 40 with a third child started tossing the child high in the air and catching him, shouting that she was letting him have a look at heaven, where he had come from. Management is similar to that for other manic psychoses, with precautions for the safety of the baby, and particular vigilance for a shift from mania to devastating depression.

ATTACHMENT BETWEEN MOTHER AND INFANT

The effect of a mother's illness of whatever type must influence profoundly the making of a secure affectional bond with her child. Caesarean section also tends to disrupt this development, and management of the mother must be coloured by consideration of the need to facilitate the 'warm, intimate, continuous relationship' between mother and baby advocated by Bowlby (1969).

Today, when, rather than assisting the mother during childbirth, midwives and others take over her body and manage her labour, it is particularly necessary to remember the basic professional duty to enable the mother-baby bond to form and the integration also of the father into the magic circle of love and dependence. The presence of the father at the birth is to be encouraged for this reason. Klaus and Kennell (1979) describe a cascade of reciprocal interactions

137

between mother and infant. A maternal sensitive period begins almost immediately after the baby is born and develops over a few days; this is the optimal time for the mother to make an affectional bond with him. The infant's attachment to mother — or a consistently reliable substitute — grows gradually over the first six to twelve months.

Drugs given to the mother during childbirth may dull the receptivity of mother and child towards each other in the earliest stages of their relationship, and should be kept to a minimum. Company and reassurance reduce the mother's need for tranquillisers. Caesarean birth, increasingly common in the United States, involves anaesthesia and amnesia for the mother. The group of Caesarean mothers in Trowell's study (1982) had no recollection of perceiving their babies until a mean of 19 hours after delivery, and although none was nursed separately, there were numerous differences in the mother's and infant's interactive behaviour for many months.

Early separation of mother and baby as a result of the latter's care in a special unit because of his medical needs arises in more than 18 per cent of cases. The effects are shown in the mother's reduced responsiveness to the child during the first two months, and increased incidence of difficult-to-interpret problems later, such as failure to thrive and non-accidental injury (see below). If an infant must be nursed in a special care unit, it is essential for the mother to be involved in the activities from the start.

Skin-to-skin contact as soon as possible after birth has been demonstrated to be of crucial importance in helping the mother-infant relationship and successful breast-feeding (De Chateau and Wilberg, 1977). Rooming-in of babies with their mothers rather than the former method of bringing them together only at feed times is associated with a better, warmer relationship over the following two years (O'Connor et al., 1977). Eye-to-eye contact between mother and child is a key factor informing a secure bond. It is sometimes lacking after Caesarean birth when a mother meets her child in the context of recovering from major abdominal surgery.

Post-Caesarean mothers, those who develop postnatal psychiatric illness and those who, on the infant's account, are separated early need continuous support, praise and encouragement to allow durable and satisfying attachments to form.

If bonding does not occur, the danger of psychosis associated with the end of a pregnancy is reduced in certain circumstances.

It is notable that post-abortion psychosis is comparatively rare: 0.3 per 1000 abortions, one-fifth of the puerperal rate (Brewer, 1978). Also somewhat surprising is the finding that there is no increase in incidence of functional psychosis after twin birth, birth of an abnormal baby or stillbirth, but perhaps large enough studies have not been made (Brockington *et al.*, 1978). Nevertheless the mothers and fathers of abnormal babies need particular consideration. The diagnosis, prognosis and sources of available help need discussing between the parents, the consultant obstetrician and the paediatrician before the mother leaves hospital.

STILLBIRTH

Stillbirth is a sad disappointment, and has been taken up with sympathy by Emanuel Lewis (1976) and later by Bourne and Lewis (1984). They suggest that the mother should hold the dead baby and keep photographs of him, and go through a funeral service. In fact full maternal bonding is normally delayed for a day or two, presumably until the baby's survival is assured (Macfarlane, 1974). To try to induce bonding artificially seems needlessly unkind, and clearly it is better to remove the mother of a stillbirth to a gynaecological ward until she leaves hospital, and to allow her to talk as much as she herself chooses about her traumatic experience.

TERMINATION OF PREGNANCY

Despite the efficacy of and improvements in contraception over the last decade, and falling birth rates, the demand for abortion continues to increase in the West. In less than one-third of cases is this related to ignorance of contraceptive techniques: clearly other factors operate. Sometimes a woman allows herself to become pregnant to test the reaction of her partner.

A simple request by the patient during the first trimester of pregnancy is all that is required to obtain a legal termination in Austria, Denmark, East Germany, France, Singapore, Sweden, Tunisia and of course the United States. For Roman Catholics abortion and contraception remain (officially) forbidden, and in many countries the moral and political dilemmas are unresolved. In the United Kingdom there are constant attempts to amend the abortion legislation: termination is permitted on grounds of potential physical or mental harm to the woman or her existing children if the pregnancy continues, or of a substantial risk that the child would be born handicapped. Two doctors must certify 'in good faith' that this is their opinion. One is often a psychiatrist. In general psychiatrists have come out in favour of widening and loosening the grounds for abortion, whereas some gynaecologists — at the sharp end — have reservations. About 100 000 legal terminations are performed annually in England and Wales (Kumar, 1983).

As already observed, there is no post-termination reaction comparable with the postpartum psychoses (see above). Indeed pre-existing depression and anxiety usually lift after abortion. Some transient feelings of guilt are frequently reported, and these may re-emerge during a subsequent wanted pregnancy. This may involve almost superstitious fears and doubts about the normality of the current foetus. Those women who become neurotically depressed months or years after a termination are usually expressing disappointment and dissatisfaction with their social and sexual situation. Broome (1984) discusses counselling immediately after termination by non-medical professionals and lay counsellors.

The liaison psychiatrist may become involved when termination has been refused and the patient is angry and upset. Some women will make private, and in the United Kingdom and some other countries illegal, arrangements. Among the remainder who go on to have the child, 50 per cent persist in wishing they had had an abortion, a substantial number suffer considerable distress, and a few are severely psychiatrically disturbed. Less than half are able to accept their situation and come to value the child (Illsley and Hall, 1976).

DANGER TO THE INFANT

Unwilling mothers and their children, especially if they are inadequately supported and socially deprived, often suffer from a string of minor physical complaints and carelessly inadequate nutrition. In these circumstances non-accidental injury — baby-battering to the media — is a high risk (see also Chapter 10). Social services input is never enough, and these mothers, nearly always young, turn to doctors as a possible source of comfort, understanding, forgiveness and practical suggestions, much as others would have gone to priests in other cultures, other centuries. These are time-consuming, important patients for whom drugs, particularly benzodiazepines, only make matters worse, leaving emphathic but unsentimental psychotherapy as the main tool together with the encouragement of as many helping agencies as possible.

As discussed, psychotic illness in a mother may lead her into trying to harm her child deliberately under the influence of delusions:

or she may neglect to feed or care for him because of psychosis, neurosis or personality problems. Obsessional ideas about injuring the child should be taken seriously. They usually fade when an accompanying depressive illness lifts. Maternal psychiatric illness, whether neurotic or psychotic, calls for particular concern for the baby. The mother must have specific treatment, support and supervision, helping her to cope with her baby so that she does not miss out on the pride and confidence of doing so; but so that the child is safe. This maximal therapeutic input is usually necessary only temporarily.

More worrying, because there is no obvious cause like maternal psychiatric illness and no time limit, is so-called non-accidental injury. This most commonly involves a child of less than two years (Margison, 1982). It is important to recognise risk factors in time to arrange an appropriate preventive and supportive safety net. Predictors of non-accidental injury are:

(1) Mother's age less than 20 at the birth of her first child.
(2) Emotional disturbance not amounting to psychiatric illness in the perinatal period.
(3) Social problems.
(4) Baby requiring admission to special care unit.
(5) Adverse comments about motherhood by the mother.
(6) Problems in pregancy: social, psychiatric or physical.
(7) Problems with labour.
(8) Separation of mother and baby after delivery.
(9) Separation during the first six months of baby's life.
(10) Illness of either mother or child during child's first year.

STERILISATION

Since laparoscopy came into common use in the late 1960s, female sterilisation has been increasingly employed as a definitive method of contraception, particularly in those over 35. The introduction of oral contraception a few years later did not lead to the expected reduction in demand for sterilisation. It may be seen as a safe and convenient contraceptive choice for those whose families are felt to be complete, and for whom the pill is contraindicated and intrauterine devices are poorly tolerated. Others with serious medical conditions may prefer to feel completely secure.

When sterilisation is considered because of the woman's mental state, psychiatric assessment is obviously necessary. Although mental impairment *per se* is no cause for sterilisation, the severely impaired and chronically psychotic, especially nymphomanic schizophrenics, may be thought suitable, on an individual basis; harm to the woman's mental state, possible harm to the foetus from medication, certain hereditary risks, for instance from Huntington's chorea, and the obvious inability of the patient to care for a child: all are factors to be weighed. The agreement in writing of the patient and discussion with concerned relatives is important. Some longstanding neurotic patients who beg for sterilisation because they are afraid of pregnancy should be regarded with caution. Their personal emotional problems are not solved by the operation and merely shift in focus, sometimes to persistent abdominal pain.

Adverse sequelae to sterilisation, either menstrual disturbance or psychiatric upset, have become less frequent over the last decade, but vary in incidence from 3 to 60 per cent (Alder, 1984). This disparity is related to the selection of patients. Those sterilised on psychiatric grounds are likely to have psychiatric problems, perhaps now blaming the sterilisation, whereas those sterilised for medical reasons are prone to understandable sadness. Patients whose current marriages show signs of instability are at risk of regretting self-chosen, irreversible sterility if divorce and remarriage ensue.

REFERENCES

Alder, E. (1984) 'Sterilization', in Broome, A. and Wallace, L. (Eds) *Psychology and Gynaecological Problems*, Tavistock, London/Methuen, New York

Alder, E.M., Cook, A., Davidson, D., West, C. and Bancroft, J. (1986) 'Hormones, Mood and Sexuality in Lactating Women', *British Journal of Psychiatry, 148*, 74-9

Areskog, B., Uddenberg, N. and Kjessler, B. (1984) 'Postnatal Emotional Balance in Women with and without Antenatal Fear of Childbirth', *Journal of Psychosomatic Research, 28*, 213-20

Backstrom, C.T., Boyle, H. and Bird, D.T. (1981) 'Persistence of Symptoms of Premenstrual Tension in Hysterectomised Women'. *British Journal of Obstetrics and Gynaecology, 880*, 530-6

Baker, A.A. (1967) *Psychiatric Disorders in Obstetrics*, Blackwell, Oxford

Barker, M.G. (1968) 'Psychiatric Illness after Hysterectomy' *British Medical Journal, 2*, 91-5

Bourne, S. and Lewis, E. (1984) 'Delayed Psychological Effects of Perinatal Death', *British Medical Journal, 289*, 147-8

Bowlby, J. (1969) *Attachment and Loss: I. Attachment*, Hogarth Press, London

Brewer, C. (1978) Chapter 5 in Sandler, M. (Ed.) *Mental Illness in Pregnancy and the Puerperium*, Oxford University Press, Oxford

Brockington, I.F. and Kumar, R. (1982) 'Drug Addiction and Psychotropic Drug Treatment during Pregnancy and Lactation, in *Motherhood and Mental Illness*, Academic Press, London

Brockington, I.F., Schofield, E.M., Donnelly, P. and Hyde, C. (1978) Chapter 6, in Sandler, M. (Ed.) *Mental Illness in Pregnancy and the Puerperium*, Oxford University Press, Oxford

Broome, A. (1984) 'Termination of Pregnancy', in Broome, A. and Wallace, L. (Eds) *Psychology and Gynaecological Problems*, Tavistock, London/Methuen, New York

Clare, A.W. (1982) *The Premenstrual Syndrome: Psychiatric Problems in Women: 3*, S.K. & F. Publications London

Clare, A.W. (1983) *Psychiatric and Social Aspects of Premenstrual Complaint*: Psychological Medicine Monograph Supplement 4, Cambridge University Press, Cambridge

Dalton, K. (1982) 'Violence and the Premenstrual Syndrome', *The Police Surgeon, 21*, 8-15

De Chateau, P. and Wilberg, B. (1977) 'Long-term Effects on Mother-Infant Behaviour of Extra Contact during the First Hour Post-partum', *Acta Psychiatrica Scandinavica, 66*, 151-61

Donovan, B.T. (1985) 'Hormones and Female Sexual Behaviour', in *Hormones and Human Behaviour*, Cambridge University Press, Cambridge

Gath, D. and Rose, N. (1985) 'Psychological Problems and Gynaecological Surgery', in Priest, R.G. (Ed.) *Psychological Disorders in Obstetrics and Gynaecology*, Butterworth, London

Illsley, R. and Hall, M.H. (1976) 'Psychosocial Aspects of Abortion: A Review of Issues and Needed Research', *Bulletin of the World Health Organization, 53*, 83-106

Jones, M.M. (1983) 'The Premenstrual Syndrome', *British Journal of Sexual Medicine, 99*, 9-11

Klaus, M.H. and Kennell, J.H. (1979) 'Early Mother-Infant Contact', *Bulletin of the Menninger Clinic, 43*, 69-78

Kumar, R. (1982) 'Neurotic Disorders', in Brockington, I.F. and Kumar, R. (Eds) *Motherhood and Mental Illness*, Academic Press, London and New York

Kumar, R. (1983) 'Reproduction and Psychiatric Disorders in Women', in Lader, M.H. (Ed.) *Mental Disorders and Somatic Illness*, Cambridge University Press

Kumar, R. and Robson, K. (1978), Chapter 4 in Sandler, M. (Ed.) *Mental Illness in Pregnancy and the Puerperium*, Oxford University Press, Oxford

Lemoine, P., Harousseau, H., Borteyru, J.P. and Menuet, J.C. (1968) 'Les enfants des parents alcooliques: anomalies observées', *Quest-Medical, 25*, 476-81

Lewis, E. (1976) 'Management of Stillbirth — Coping with an Unreality', *Lancet, 2*, 619-20

Macfarlane, A. (1974) 'If a Smile is So Important', *New Scientist, 62*, 164-6

Marcé, L.V. (1858) 'Traité de la folie des femmes enceintes', quoted in Baker, A.A. (1967) *Psychiatric Disorders in Obstetrics*, Blackwell, Oxford

Margison, F. (1982) 'The Pathology of the Mother-Child Relationship', in Brockington, I.F. and Kumar, R. (Eds) *Motherhood and Mental Illness*,

Academic Press, London and New York

Mattsson, B. and Schoultz, B.V. (1974) 'A Comparison between Lithium, Placebo and Diuretic in Premenstrual Tension', *Acta Psychiatrica Scandinavica; Supplement, 255,* 75-84

O'Connor, S.W., Vietze, P.M., Hopkins, J.B. and Altmeier, W.A. (1977) 'Post-partum Extended Maternal-Infant Contact: Subsequent Mothering and Child Health', *Pediatric Research, 11,* 380-90

Oppenheim, G.B. (1985) 'Psychological Disorders in Pregnancy', in Priest, R.G. (Ed.) *Psychological Disorders in Obstetrics and Gynaecology,* Butterworths, London

Paykel, E.S., Emms, E.M., Fletcher, G.A. and Rassaby, E.S. (1980) 'Life Events and Social Support in Puerperal Depression', *British Journal of Psychiatry, 136,* 339-46

Pitt, B. (1973) 'Maternity Blues', *British Journal of Psychiatry, 122,* 431-3

Pitt, B. (1985) 'The Puerperium', in Priest, R.G. (Ed.) *Psychological Disorders in Obstetrics and Gynaecology,* Butterworths, London

Reid, R.L. and Yen, S.S.C. (1981) 'Premenstrual Syndrome', *American Journal of Obstetrics and Gynaecology, 139,* 85

Sandler, M. (Ed.) (1978) *Mental Illness in Pregnancy and the Puerperium,* Oxford University Press, Oxford

Slade, P. (1984) 'Premenstrual Emotional Changes in Normal Women: Fact or Fiction?', *Journal of Psychosomatic Research, 28,* 1-7

Stein, G. (1982) 'The Maternity Blues', in Brockington, I.F.L and Kumar, R. (Eds) *Motherhood and Mental Illness,* Academic Press, London and New York

Trowell, J. (1982) 'Effects of Obstetric Management in the Mother-Child Relationship', in Parkes, C.M. and Stevenson-Hinde, J. (Eds) *The Place of Attachment in Human Behaviour,* Tavistock, London/Methuen, New York

Turpin, T.J. and Heath, D.A. (1979) 'The Link between Hysterectomy and Depression', *Canadian Journal of Psychiatry, 24,* 247-54

Van Keep, P.A. and Lehert, P. (1981) *The Premenstrual Syndrome,* MTP Press, Lancaster

Whitlock, F.A., (1982) Chapter 9 in *Symptomatic Affective Disorders.* Academic Press, Sydney.

World Health Organization (1978) *Mental Disorders: Glossary and Guide to their Classification in Accordance with the Ninth Revision of the International Classification of Disease,* WHO, Geneva

9

Liaison in Endocrine and Metabolic Problems

The major systems of communication within the body are neural and endocrine. In contrast to the instantaneous, transient action of neurotransmitters, hormones, when their message is decoded at the appropriate site, influence cellular metabolism over minutes, hours, days or longer. The hypothalamus and adjacent parts of the brain have an important regulatory function over both systems and are concerned with temperature control, the sleep-wake cycle, eating, drinking, sexual activity and aggression. They are intimately involved on a two-way basis through the limbic system with emotional status. This in turn is influenced by cognitive factors: the appraisal of internal and external perceptions in the light of experience and memory. Inevitably endocrine and metabolic disturbances produce psychiatric and behavioural symptoms, and psychological upsets impinge upon endocrine equilibrium.

Differentiation between predominantly psychiatric and basically endocrine disorders is facilitated by modern laboratory techniques. Hormone levels may now be rapidly, accurately and economically estimated from small samples of body fluid by radioimmunoassay. The cerebral mechanisms by which hormonal abnormalities induce psychological changes are not fully understood; the effects lack the specificity sought by psychoanalysts (Dunbar, 1954). Manfred Bleuler (1954) described a general endocrine psychosyndrome comprising fluctuant behavioural and emotional features, including moodiness, anxiety, irritability and childishness, and somatic symptoms with psychological connotations, such as impotence, lethargy and altered appearance.

PSYCHIATRIC COMPLICATIONS OF ENDOCRINE DISEASE

The earliest indication of these may be changes in personality or behaviour, and difficulties in coping, which may indeed comprise the initial presentation of the illness. Later manifestations include maladaptive ways of responding to the disorder, including deviant illness behaviour such as non-compliance with medical management, active denial of disability, or regressive dependence. Bleuler's endocrine psychosyndrome may develop, or a symptomatic functional psychiatric syndrome of schizophreniform, paranoid or affective type. Organic brain syndromes may arise, ranging from coma to delirium, the amnestic syndrome and other circumscribed organic states, hallucinosis or a progressive dementing process (after Beumont, 1979). The pathogenesis of psychiatric symptomatology in endocrine disease resides in a variety of overlapping factors: brain damage in temporary metabolic disruption; altered sensory input and feedback, including body image; distortions of perceived meaning; upset sleep-wake rhythm; and the patient's inability to fulfil the demands of his social role. The relative importance of these factors in producing symptoms depends on the interplay between somatic factors including the severity of the disease and such host characteristics as age, sex, individual vulnerability, and environmental features, especially adequacy of interpersonal relationships and support system.

In the evaluation of aetiology and the making of a treatment plan in endocrine disease, equal attention must be given to psychological and social aspects as to physical, neurological and laboratory examination. Liaison is an integral part of assessment (Sachar, 1975; Popkin and Mackenzie, 1980).

SPECIFIC ENDOCRINE SYNDROMES

Acromegaly

Acromegaly affects either sex and usually appears in early or middle adult life. Excessive growth hormone production from a slow-growing acidophil cell pituitary tumour causes characteristic changes in face, hands and feet. Other features are excessive sweating, loss of libido or disturbed menses, and headaches. Later manifestations are impaired visual fields and symptoms of raised intracranial pressure. Diabetes mellitus, carpal tunnel syndrome, hypertension and arthritis may also develop. In spite of disfigurement and sexual symptoms which might be upsetting, gross psychiatric disorder is rare in acromegaly. The patient is often unduly passive and apathetic; he may be mildly depressed or euphoric and his memory may be impaired.

Medical treatment, for instance with bromocriptine, or surgery leads to a slow improvement of physical symptoms. A stimulating antidepressant such as clomipramine, imipramine or tranylcypromine may be helpful for the apathetic patient. Clomipramine — in the UK only — or imipramine may be given in dosage of 30-150 mg daily, in divided doses; tranylcypromine, and MAOI, in the range 10-30 mg, divided, before 4 pm.

Panhypopituitarism

Symptoms of hormonal insufficiency are unusual after hypophysectomy or irradiation because of routine, prompt institution of replacement therapy. Other causes of more or less generalised hypopituitarism are pressure from, for instance, a craniopharyngioma or chromophobe adenoma; infarction, sometimes from cerebrovascular disease; head injury; sarcoidosis; meningitis or — rarely nowadays — postpartum necrosis. There is a secretory failure, which may be uneven, of adrenocorticotrophic hormone (ACTH), thyroid-stimulating hormone, gonadotrophin and growth hormone.

Presentation depends on the age of the patient. Short stature and failure of puberty in children arouse concern, and in middle age the onset is insidious, with a cluster of symptoms which may be considered neurotic initially. Lethargy, weakness, loss of libido, poor memory, intolerance to cold, anxiety and depression are associated with somatic features: pallor, thin dry skin, impotence or amenorrhoea, genital atrophy and diminution of body hair and beard. The effects are like those of ageing, inappropriately early. There may be marked weight loss, which used to cause confusion between postpartum hypopituitarism and anorexia nervosa. In the latter the patient is alert, often lively and shows an overriding determination to keep the weight below normal. The features of Bleuler's endocrine psychosyndrome are well displayed in panhypopituitarism, with loss of initiative and memory impairment as early symptoms.

Treatment of the underlying cause where possible must be accompanied by hormone substitution therapy with cortisone and thyroxine together, and in some young patients appropriate sex steroids. It is important not to give thyroxine without cortisone, or a hypoadrenal crisis may be provoked. In vulnerable patients a paranoid or euphoric state may be precipitated by too high and too rapid a dosage of cortisone. An acute organic psychosis may arise and persist for several weeks following hypopituitary coma or other physical crisis. General physical and psychological symptoms both subside with hormonal treatment, with apathy the last to recover. Psychotic symptoms may require reducing doses of haloperidol over a few days or weeks only. Of course hypopituitarism provides no protection from coincidental psychiatric disorder, for instance schizophrenia, which requires treatment in its own right.

Short stature

Organically caused failure of pituitary function impairs structural growth through deficiency of growth hormone. Psychologically the patient suffers the disadvantages of being babied, and is likely to become dependent, over-conforming, and unable to express aggression. Puberty sharpens the adjustment problems, and even more emotional upset may occur in response to rapid hormone-induced growth. Loss of privileges and indulgence because of small size may be regretted. Acting out and psychotic episodes are conspicuously absent in these patients (Money and Pollitt, 1966).

> *Case*: J.V., 16, developed a variant of anorexia nervosa in an attempt to keep his height low: he rigorously avoided proteinous foods. He had the appearance of a boy of ten or eleven and enjoyed travel and other facilities accorded to children, and was in demand as a cox.

Reversible somatotrophin deficiency

Reversible somatotrophin deficiency (psychosocial dwarfism) results from suppression of growth hormone release from severe emotional and environmental deprivation. Bone age is reduced, intellectual development retarded, and sleep impaired. Bizarre behaviour, such as eating garbage, polydipsia, and tantrums alternating with apathy, is common. All the symptoms including physical and mental retardation recover on removal to a different environment. The administration of propranolol reverses the growth hormone deficiency. Family therapy must precede and accompany the child's return home (Wolff and Money, 1973). Other causes of short stature include malnutrition, chronic infection, hypothyroidism, Turner's syndrome, and achondroplasia. In these, normal or high-level growth hormone response is found. 'Failure to thrive' in an infant who typically does well in hospital is an early warning of emotional deprivation.

Diabetes insipidus

This is the only recognised deficiency syndrome associated with the posterior pituitary, and is due to lack of antidiuretic hormone (ADH). Characteristic symptoms are apathy, dysphoria, loss of libido, and increased desire for sleep, with polydipsia, polyuria and an outflow of 5-10 litres daily. There may be an obvious cause of damage in the region of pituitary fossa or none may be evident. Nephrogenic diabetes insipidus depends on unresponsiveness of the nephron to the action of ADH and may be hereditary, when it is usually associated with infantilism and mental impairment, or due to the effect of lithium therapy, frequently used in manic depression. Diabetes mellitus and chronic renal failure also require exclusion, but the condition most likely to involve the liaison psychiatrist is *compulsive water drinking*, a neurotic disorder with overtones of hysterical gain. The water deprivation test is useful is assessing ADH deficiency although direct assay is available in some laboratories. The administration of an ADH analogue produces immediate, dramatic improvement in diabetes insipidus. In compulsive water drinking, polydipsia continues, producing water intoxication with nausea, vomiting, headache and confusion but seldom oedema. Treatment of compulsive water drinking involves painstaking history taking and psychotherapeutic and psychosocial support. There is occasionally a depressive element calling for drug treatment with, for instance amitriptyline or doxepin in 50-200 mg daily dosage for either. ADH secretion is enhanced by physical or mental stress, inappropriate secretion from, for instance, lung disease, nicotine, morphine and tricyclic antidepressants (Donovan, 1985).

Hypercortisolism: Cushing's syndrome

This condition may arise spontaneously or iatrogenically. There may be primary dysfunction of the adrenal cortex, usually from a benign or malignant tumour, or adrenocortical hyperplasia may be secondary to overproduction of ACTH in the pituitary: often from basophil microadenomata. This type is true Cushing's disease and accounts for 80 per cent of cases. Ectopic ACTH secretion in a tumour such as oat-cell bronchial carcinoma or carcinoid may produce a similar syndrome.

Onset is variable and insidious in naturally occurring

hypercortisolism. Symptoms include obesity with buffalo distribution, striae, red moon-shaped face, hirsuities, easy bruising, muscular weakness, and loss of libido with oligomenorrhoea or impotence. Hypertension and disturbed glucose metabolism also occur. Women are affected five times more often than men, and psychiatric symptoms are likely to present before the clinical picture is clearly recognisable. In these cases a psychiatric opinion may be sought early. Emotional overreactivity is common in Cushingoid patients even without formal psychiatric illness. The commonest disorder is depression. This may be of the neurotic type with tearfulness, irritability and hypochondriasis. Altered appearance, with obscuring of personal identifying characteristics in face and form, and of gender markings, can have a profound effect on the patient's self-image and confidence. Psychotic depression, a more directly metabolic effect, is also common and carries a high risk of suicide. Less commonly a euphoric or manic state or a mixed paranoid psychosis develops, or a frank acute organic brain syndrome with disorientation.

> *Case*: Mrs P.L., 45, while undergoing inpatient investigation, became increasingly angry, noisy and overactive during the course of a few days, accusing the nursing staff of stealing and her husband of rampant infidelity. She saw car headlights coming towards her in the hospital corridor. She had a pituitary tumour.

Patients with Cushing's syndrome associated with malignant lung tumour rarely show a typical picture of hypercortisolism but but rapidly progressive weight loss, weakness, oedema and pigmentation.

Diagnosis in hypocortisolism by the dexamethasone suppression test and related others may be in question because of positive results found in depression, weight loss, alcoholism and acute use of some drugs.

Treatment. Definitive treatment of hypercortisolism either surgically or medically including metyrapone suppression, usually relieves both physical and psychiatric symptoms in the long term. In a proportion of cases the patient is too distressed, too disruptive or too suicidal to await this outcome and requires urgent symptomatic psychiatric treatment. Haloperidol by any route is the main standby in delirious, manic or acute paranoid states, with clomipramine or amitriptyline combined with 1 mg doses of trifluoperazine in the severely depressed. Constant nursing observation and if necessary sedation is required while a suicidal risk remains. Assessment of this depends on the patient's feelings of guilt, self-blame or worthlessness and persecutory or nihilistic delusions.

Iatrogenic hyperecortisolism

Systemic or topical corticosteroid administration may lead to psychological disturbance at any stage in treatment, even within a few hours of the first dose, although a time lag of a week is likelier. The psychiatric reaction is to some extent dose-related and may be precipitated by potassium depletion after diuretics. It may take any form or change back and forth from one to another: Hall's 'spectrum psychosis' (Hall *et al.*, 1979). Prange *et al.* (1975) found euphoria the most frequent reaction. Multiple sclerosis, rheumatoid arthritis and systemic lupus erythematosis are all disorders frequently associated with affective disturbance in their own right, and in which steroids are often prescribed. The need for the continuation of steroids must be balanced against the psychiatric upset and psychotropics exhibited accordingly. Neuroleptic treatment is usually effective, but in depressed patients tricyclics alone sometimes worsen the disturbance: the physician should be warned of this.

Nelson's syndrome

Nelson's syndrome is a late result of adrenalectomy with an enlarging pituitary tumour and hypersecretion of ACTH and melanocyte-stimulating hormone (MSH), with intense pigmentation. Psychiatric disturbances are surprisingly infrequent and when they present do so as a neurotic reaction to the change in appearance.

> *Case*: Mr L., 39, had been good looking and fair skinned when he married. His wife deserted him when he developed Nelson's syndrome. The neighbours had begun asking Mrs L. about her husband's country of origin. Mr. L. became reactively depressed and attempted suicide by overdosage.

Pseudo-Cushing's syndrome

Chronic alcohol excess may induce raised cortisol levels and all the manifestations of Cushing's syndrome. These do not persist, however, and there is evidence of alcohol abuse. Depression is common in these cases and needs treating as well as the alcoholism. Simple obesity may be mistaken for hypercortisolism but the history and diagnostic tests differentiate between the two.

Chronic adrenocortical insufficiency: Addison's disease

This comprises lack of cortisol and aldosterone secretion and the primary disease results from autoimmune or tuberculous damage to the adrenal cortex. A secondary chronic form results from hypothalamo-pituitary failure. As in Cushing's syndrome, onset in Addison's disease is typically gradual, and physical symptoms are frequently preceded by psychological: fatigue, apathy, low libido, mild cognitive impairment, poverty of thought and lack of initiative in a setting of general depression, which is unresponsive to psychiatric treatment. Psychiatric symptoms occur in at least two-thirds of patients, with depression in 45 per cent. When the disease has been present for several years, frankly organic brain syndromes may emerge.

Physical symptoms to look for are anorexia, nausea, vomiting and weight loss; back or abdominal pain, hypotension and syncope; and slatey-brown pigmentation on exposed areas of skin, those subject to pressure, and inside the mouth. Electrolyte abnormalities, diffuse electroencephalographic changes with high-amplitude slow waves, and specific laboratory tests (including tetracosactrin challenge) clarify the diagnosis. Occasionally such patients are misdiagnosed as suffering from anorexia nervosa with pigmentation from hypercarotenaemia.

Addisonian crises in which the patient is acutely ill, hypotensive and hypoglycaemic may be precipitated by trauma including surgery, infection or the administration of thyroxine with too little cortisone in hypopituitary states. The psychiatric picture is of anxiety quickly giving way to an acute organic reaction and even coma. In Addison's disease, replacement therapy is required lifelong with cortisone and also fludrocortisone if aldosterone deficiency is marked. Symptoms of apathy and depression and those of crisis usually clear with this treatment, but a steroid psychosis is not uncommon and pigmentation tends to persist (Whitlock, 1982).

Phaeochromocytoma

Recurrent attacks of acute anxiety, headache and hypertension in a young adult should arouse suspicion of this rare tumour, which secretes excessive amounts of adrenaline and noradrenaline. In 90 per cent of cases the tumour is in the adrenal medulla; in the rest it — or they — may be anywhere along the sympathetic chain. Diagnosis depends on laboratory studies of plasma or 24-hour urine. Treatment is surgical but there may be technical problems in stabilising the blood pressure for this, or if more than one tumour exists but is undiscovered. There is in any case often a need to calm the patient's distress and reduce his blood pressure: beta-blockers and benzodiazepine anxiolytics are useful in addition to phenoxybenzamine, 10 mg twice daily increasing as needed. Propranolol must be introduced after phenoxybenzamine: doses of 10 mg three times daily may be given chronically, doubling in the run up to surgery. Diazepam 5-10 mg twice daily may be started at any time.

Thyroid disorders

These are common and nearly always involve prominent psychiatric symptoms. There is a genetic element in 50 per cent of cases and women are affected far more often than men. Hyperthyroidism is four times as common in females, typically in early adult life: the key mood is anxiety. Hypothyroidism is ten times commoner in women and mainly affects the middle-aged and elderly: the prevailing mood is depressive.

Hyperthyroid patients are insomniac and irritable, and easily become quarrelsome and uncooperative with treatment: this may involve the psychiatrist. Other features are weight loss with good appetite; exhaustion but continuing restlessness; impaired memory and concentration; intolerance to heat; tremor and tachycardia even in sleep; and sweating. The thyroid gland is enlarged, smoothly or irregularly; tendon reflexes are rapid and brisk; and even in the absence of gross signs the eyes are wide open: 'the thyroid glitter'. Occasionally in the older patient the 'apathetic' variety of hyperthyroidism may arise: lassitude and cardiovascular symptoms, such as atrial fibrillation or congestive failure, are the hallmarks.

Diagnosis is clinched by biochemical tests: it should be noted that a raised thyroxine level may be due to increase of binding globulin, as in pregnancy, with the oral contraceptive or other oestrogen-containing pills, clofibrate and phenothiazines. The free thyroxine index (FTI) corrects for this.

Treatment. Improvement in both physical and psychological

symptoms is delayed for 4-6 weeks after starting definitive treatment with carbimazole; with radioiodine the time scale is measured in months. Surgery, if undertaken, is preceded by carbimazole treatment. Thus there always remains a period in which symptomatic treatment is required: with a beta-blocker (e.g. propranolol 40 mg TDS) and an anxiolytic, e.g. lorazepam 1 mg or alprazolam 0.5 mg two or three times daily. If there is a troublesome paranoid element, trifluoperazine 1 mg b.d. is useful. Exophthalmos, if present, tends to persist, disappointingly.

Thyroid storm. A sudden, severe acute exacerbation of hyperthyroidism may bring on a wild delirious state, with fear and paranoid ideation prominent, which shifts towards coma ominously. Urgent intravenous therapy is called for with intravenous propanolol, 5 mg, and intravenous chlorpromazine in dosage just sufficient for sedation: 25-75 mg, slowly. This is a dangerous condition and the effects of medication need to be rapid and observable.

Hypothyroidism. This can arise *in utero* or early life but is commonest in middle adulthood, due to autoimmune disease or as an end-result of Hashimoto's thyroiditis. It may be secondary to pituitary failure in panhypopituitarism, long-term lithium prophylaxis in manic depression, following thyroidectomy or after radioiodine therapy for hyperthyroidism. Almost any psychiatric disturbance may be associated with the hypothyroid state, but a typical presentaation is in a woman of 40-60 with any of a cluster of neurotic-seeming symptoms: mental and physical retardation and lethargy, generalised mild misery, poor memory, slight weight increase and feeling the cold. More obviously physical symptoms are hair loss, including the outer third of the eyebrows; parchment-pale, coarse, dry skin; puffiness under the eyes and occasionally oedema elsewhere; hoarse voice, menstrual irregularities; fluctuant Eustachian deafness; carpal tunnel syndrome; and slow reflexes. The electrocardiogram may show low-voltage complexes and a flat or inverted T-wave;

In the elderly, clinical findings may antedate positive biochemical tests (Cropper, 1973). In some of these, cognitive deficits may be sufficiently severe to raise the question of dementia. However, only 1 in 100 psychogeriatric admissions were found to be hypothyroid by Henschke and Pain (1977). A paranoid illness resembling schizophrenia or an acute organic syndrome — Asher's (1949) 'myxoedematous madness' — may also occur in hypothyroidism. In a conference on myxoedema in 1888 it was reported that one-third of ference on myxoedema in 1888 it was reported that one-third of patients had hallucinations and delusions: with earlier diagnosis and better treatment these are now a rarity (Beumont, 1979).

Case: Miss A.H., a slim woman of 34, was admitted to a psychiatric ward with auditory hallucinations and delusions that darts were being shot at her. She also mentioned in passing that her body felt like lead. The correct diagnosis was made only after she suffered a cardiac arrest in reaction to thioridazine (Gomez and Scott, 1980).

Treatment: a starting dose of 0.05 mg or in the very elderly 0.025 mg thyroxine daily is increased as necessary, probably to 0.2 mg daily. Apart from cardiac complications, too rapid an introduction of full doses can induce a thyroid crisis. Since thyroxine is slow-acting, it need be taken only once in the 24 hours — but life-long. Symptomatic recovery lags behind the biochemical, maybe for weeks, and tricyclic antidepressants and/or ECT work well in depressed patients meanwhile (Gibbons, 1983). In paranoid cases haloperidol is the safest tranquilliser in view of the risk of inducing cardiac complications or of hypothermic hypothyroid coma. In the latter case the physician must give, urgently, hydrocortisone and intravenous triiodothyronine.

Cretinism

Hypothyroid babies have coarse features, a hoarse cry and are retarded. Prognosis for full intellectual recovery is poor in congenital cases but prompt treatment is vital in all. These children are said to be awkward and suspicious: perhaps a function of other people's reactions to them (Beumont, 1979).

Hyper- and hypocalcaemia

Calcium is the most prevalent cation in the body, and normal serum levels lie within a narrow range: 2.3–2.6 mmol/1. Excessive secretion of parathyroid hormone, as in adenoma of the gland, leads to hypercalcaemia, as does excessive administration of vitamin D. It is important for the liaison psychiatrist to remember also that renal and bronchial carcinomas in particular, with or without bony metastases, sarcoidosis and immobilisation in cases of Paget's disease (because of active bone metabolism), also induce raised calcium levels. Calcium is thought to deplete noradrenaline so it is unsurprising that both apathy and depression are frequently found with hypercalcaemia (Lishman,

1978). Intellectual fall-off and paranoid organic psychoses are likely at higher levels. Physical symptoms are vague: anorexia, weakness, constipation, thirst and polyuria. Accurate organic diagnosis is the main essential: the psychiatrist may help with this and with symptomatic treatment. Magnesium levels are often disturbed in conjunction with calcium abnormalities, and low magnesium is usually accompanied by low mood.

Hypocalcaemia most often results from damage to the parathyroid glands during laryngeal or thyroid surgery, but may be nutritional and is described in advanced breast cancer (Webb and Gehi, 1980). Reduced calcium levels lead to perioral paraesthesiae, neuromuscular irritability and even epileptic convulsions. The prevailing mood is anxiety, and if this is associated with even a minor degree of hyperventilation (which reduces ionised calcium), dramatic symptoms result. In severe hypocalcaemia, paranoid psychoses, acute organic brain syndromes, and curious states of rigidity and mutism may test the diagnostic acumen of the liaison psychiatrist. If neuroleptics are given symptomatically, it should be remembered that dystonic reactions are particularly likely to occur in these patients.

Diabetes mellitus

A spontaneous deficiency of insulin occurs in this disease, which comprises a juvenile, often severe, type and a milder later-onset type with a hereditary factor. It may also be secondary to alcoholic or other chronic pancreatic disease. The earliest symptoms of diabetes may come over as neurotic: fatigue, polyuria, blurred vision, or merely impotence; or the disease may present explosively with ketoacidosis and delirium or hyperosmolar coma. In spite of disruption to their lives including school activities, diabetic children are surprisingly resilient until puberty when resentment at being 'different', with reproductive connotations, may call for counselling. The parents often show more emotional disturbance than the patient: depression in the mother and marital conflicts are common (Turk and Speers, 1983).

Emotional and physical stress may effect diabetes adversely but not in any consistent way. Problems over compliance with treatment are more likely than psychiatric symptoms in diabetics. Adolescents and neurotic young adults, usually women, occasionally omit or overdose with insulin as a suicidal threat or serious attempt usually in reaction to a relationship crisis, and insulin is a favourite overdose drug among doctors and nurses. Diabetes mellitus and anorexia nervosa sometimes occur together, probably not more often than by chance with two relatively common disorders. In the combination diabetes may run dangerously out of control. Establishing rapport with both physician and psychiatrist is needed, with a safety net of psychotherapeutic support.

In later life the effects of atheroma, hypertension and recurrent episodes of accidental neuroglycopenia take their toll, and a chronic, progressive, organic brain syndrome emerges. Depression is a not uncommon reaction to this in the early stages. Patients whose diabetes is secondary to pancreatic carcinoma or chronic pancreatitis are also likely to be depressed.

Diabetic coma may be preceded by delirium and requires urgent medical treatment.

Hypoglycaemia

This is defined arbitrarily as a blood glucose level below 2.2 mmol/l. What is relevant to symptomatology is neuroglycopenia: an insufficiency of available glucose to maintain normal cerebral functioning. It is accompanied by an outflow of adrenaline which acts to raise blood sugar, inhibits its use outside the central nervous system, and mobilises fatty acids as fuel elsewhere. Growth hormone has a similar but less instantaneous effect and its increase is part of the adaptive response in anorexia nervosa and other starvation.

Acute neuroglycopenia occurs after accidental or factitious insulin overdosage. Vague unease gives way to anxiety, depersonalisation and disinhibition. The patient is flushed, sweating, restless and unsteady; he feels hungry. Coma follows unless glucose is given urgently.

Chronic neuroglycopenia has an insidious onset with deterioration of personality, memory and general intellectual functioning, and perhaps a paranoid psychosis. There may be acute episodes, not associated with eating. The cause is likely to be insulinoma (prevalence one in 1 000 000), but pituitary, adrenal, thyroid or hepatic insufficiency may incidentally involve neuroglycopenia (Marks, 1966).

Alcohol-induced neuroglycopenia comes on 6-36 hours after moderate to heavy alcohol intake without appreciable food. The patient is not necessarily generally malnourished. He is likely to be found comatose and may be regarded as 'sleeping it off'. Intravenous glucose 25 mg as 50 per cent dextrose solution and cortisone 25 mg if there is no response to two 25 mg doses of dextrose are needed urgently:

this condition carries a high mortality.

Case: Mr B., 32, was an inpatient over the weekend awaiting elective minor surgery. He went out just before lunch and returned in the late afternoon having drunk six pints of beer. He went to bed and slept for a few hours. At 10.00 p.m. he got up, had a cup of tea and chatted up the nurses in a somewhat disinhibited way before going to sleep. He was dead next morning. Post-mortem drew blank.

Post-gastrectomy hypoglycaemia appears to depend on the rapid transit of food to the jejunum and a steep rise in blood sugar inducing excessive insulin release. A dietary shift away from easily absorbed carbohydrate may help. Understandably, some patients with neurotic problems are particularly disabled by this condition.

Spontaneous reactive hypoglycaemia, a hypoglycaemic rebound to a large dose of oral carbohydrate, is a normal phenomenon not associated with symptoms of neuroglycopenia. It may be that some patients suffer postprandial weakness, anxiety and general emotional distress because of hypoglycaemia, but Ford *et al*. (1976) and Marks (1975) believe, as the result of their studies, that patients with a psychiatric illness may have their symptoms attributed erroneously to incidental glucose-tolerance-test findings, and that the real danger to the patient is that a depressive illness will pass untreated.

Menopause

Ovarian function begins to decline from around 40, and fertility diminishes. Final failure of appreciable ovarian oestrogen secretion with cessation of the menses occurs relatively suddenly eight to ten years later. Oestrogen production is maintained at a new level through the adrenals. Up to 90 per cent of menopausal women experience 'hot flushes', sometimes over many months, due to vasomotor instability associated with the abrupt drop in oestrogen. Vaginitis, which may cause irritation and dyspareunia, also results from oestrogen deficiency in some patients. A wide range of general and emotional symptoms is also ascribed to the menopause by some women, including tiredness, depression, insomnia, irritability, impaired concentration, headaches and tension. Such symptoms and hypochondriacal concern over bodily changes are common in the perimenopausal period, particularly in those who have had previous psychiatric problems.

While vaginitis is appropriately treated with an oestrogen cream, and hot flushes with a limited period on systemic oestrogens, emotional distress and neurotic symptoms are unlikely to be endocrine in origin, and should not be treated by hormone replacement therapy (HRT) (Ballinger, 1976, 1985). Support and in some case psychotropic medication are more appropriate.

Eating disorders

Both obesity and persistent underweight are usually the result of a primary eating disorder (Figure 9.1). The causes of secondary weight change must also be considered.

Figure 9.1: Eating Disorders Continuum

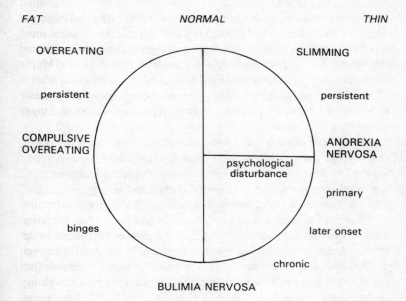

Obesity

Endocrine causes include hypothyroidism, Cushing's syndrome and failure of metabolic readjustment after pregnancy. Alcohol excess — 'beer tummy' — may also lead to fat deposition and a fatty liver. Stopping smoking raises the set level for blood glucose apparently permanently, and causes some weight gain. Drugs associated with weight gain, through increasing appetite, are cannabis, sodium valproate, phenothiazines especially chlorpromazine, and tricyclic antidepressants. The latter also restore faulty glucose utilisation in depression. MAOIs sometimes induce hypoglycaemia and hence stimulate hunger. In early hypomania, eating, like other activities, may be excessive and cause weight gain, and some tense or depressed patients find relief in constant eating. None of these conditions leads to massive obesity.

Primary overeating may be a simple matter of steady habitual intake in excess of need, or a compulsion to eat too much which may come in bouts, as bulimia nervosa but with inadequate disposal of the nutritional load. Marked bingeing occurs in 51 per cent of patients complaining of obesity, moderate bingeing in 26 per cent. One form is reactive hyperphagia: the patient starves all day but by evening she is tired and her resolve relaxes: she eats ravenously in the evening and night.

Predisposing factors include female sex; family trait and expectation of fatness; family eating habits (equally applicable to adoptees), in which tastes are trained towards cheeseburgers, chips and chocolate; the youngest or only and particularly precious child; little exercise for whatever reason; constitutional failure of the normal switch-off of endorphins when eating begins; unsatisfactory relationships and dysphoric feelings of anger, anxiety or unhappiness — not to the level of psychiatric illness.

Effects of obesity are both physical, with cardiovascular, respiratory, gynaecological and joint complications, and psychological. At 50 per cent overweight, arousal is reduced including anxiety or other emotional distress; sexual interest and activity are reduced and this may be a relief rather than a cause for regret.

Treatment is aimed at physiological disruption so that the body uses its own fat for fuel, followed by long-term restructured eating habits. A diet with adequate protein and fibre but a calorific value of 300-400 kcal is needed, with regular exercise. Behavioural manoeuvres may help some patients. Drugs are unhelpful except for replacement dosage of triiodothyronine (75 mcg daily) if the pulse rate falls below 60, indicating slowed metabolism. Regular supportive psychotherapy, individual or group, is essential for at least two years. Gastric clipping, by-pass, jaw wiring and nylon belts help some patients, but cannot be recommended generally. Appetite suppressants, thyroid hormones (except as above), diuretics and laxatives are contraindicated.

The effects of weight loss to be expected are (transiently) weakness, headache, craving for food, and with appreciable weight loss amenor-rhoea, insomnia and hyperactivity. Anxiety and depression may be felt more acutely until observable success provides a reward.

Persistent underweight

This may be secondary to hyperthyroidism, Addison's disease, hypopituitarism, malignancy and any chronic systemic disease. Acute upsets may cause temporary anorexia, but this may be more persis-tent in depression or schizophrenia with food-related delusions. Nicotine, caffeine, opiates and amphetamine analogues also reduce appetite.

Anorexia nervosa

This implies a wilful refusal to maintain normal weight, a weight loss of more than 10 per cent and amenorrhoea (Dally and Gomez, 1979). Females are affected nearly 20 times as often as males. There are several varieties: *primary*, set off by puberty, including 4 per cent arising before menarche; *secondary*, set off by threat of sexual respon-sibility, usually in those of 19 or more; and *anorexia tardive*, which is a method of manipulating husband or children often after age 45. This form is increasing in incidence.

Predisposing factors include a culture in which extreme thin-ness is highly regarded; a food-conscious, often middle-class family; the family attitude that a good child gives, but asks for nothing; parents who expect excellence but do nothing to underpin this; vul-nerable adolescence; and a particular need to control weight as in modelling or ballet. Precipitants include the normal increase in weight from ages 13-17 which subsides naturally by 18; examinations and fear of failure; fortuitous weight loss from, for instance, glandular fever; depression or death of mother; and perceived threat associated with sexuality.

Perpetuating factors include an attempt to recapture the early 'high'; beta-endophins are increased in early starvation and with exercise, giving a feeling of clear-headedness, energy and well-being which is immediately doused by eating. Others are the alarming preoccupa-tion with food — a side-effect of starvation; bloating from delayed gastric emptying; gratifying changes in family attitudes; unresolved predisposing factors; and obsessionality, which is enhanced by weight loss in anyone.

Effects of starvation include: acrocyanosis; increased body hair; reduction in T3, balanced by reverse T3 production; increased growth hormone; reduced luteinising hormone; decreased insulin sensitivity;

161

impaired thermoregulation, high plasma cortisol at 4 a.m. (and a positive dexamethasone test); reduced noradrenaline turnover; hyperactivity, irritability and depression; and reduced powers of concentration and conceptualisation.

Treatment: restoration of weight with adequate food intake aided by a reward behavioural system is essential for survival and also to allow psychotherapeutic progress from purely supportive to gently insightful, helping the patient to sense and to strengthen her own individuality. Except in mild cases, psychotherapy will need to be continued for at least two years. Family therapy is also useful in the first few months. Occasionally, if the patient is extremely distressed and her behaviour violently disturbed, chlorpromazine may be given initially in sufficient dosage to calm the patient, probably 25 mg doses repeated three to four times in the day if necessary will be enough. Larger doses increase the small risk of a *grand mal* convulsion and should be kept to the minimum consistent with management. Other medication — naloxone, cyproheptadine, sodium valproate, zinc, bromocriptine, lithium and antidepressants — all are of little use. Anorectics whose disorder is institutionalised in marriage, including the older group with anorexia tardive, are more likely to vomit or use laxatives deceptively, even in hospital. These patients do not respond to the simple refeed and reward system used in primary cases but require more intensive individual and couples therapy. Occasionally the older patients are depressed in a neurotic sense and may be helped a little by Parstelin (tranylcypromine 10 mg with trifluoperazine 1 mg which may have to be given as separate tablets in the US) or amitriptyline. The MAOI should be given once or twice in the early part of the day; amitriptyline in these patients is best given at night as 25-75 mg. These patients often cause the physicians anxiety in case malignancy has been missed. Treatment is often unsuccessful since there is nothing the psychiatrist or physician can offer that is as gratifying as the family response to the illness.

Bulimia nervosa

This condition was so-named by Russell (1979) as 'an ominous variant of anorexia nervosa'. It comprises preoccupation with food, including episodes of gorging. There is a morbid dread of fatness and the patient makes desperate attempts to control her nutrition by vomiting, purging and/or episodes of starvation. Those with hysterical personalities tend to vomit, causing loss of nutrition and loss of potassium. Those of more obsessional temperament try starving or laxative abuse: the latter causing loss of fluid not fat, and of potassium. Cardiac dysrhythmias may arise from disrupted noradrenaline turnover and low potassium levels. The periods may continue or become irregular.

Tension and depression are common in bulimia nervosa, sometimes leading to overdosing. Personal relationships are upset and unsatisfactory, and treatment aims at improving communication while gradually gaining control of eating behaviour. The patient should keep a diary of her feelings towards key figures in her life, recorded immediately before eating, vomiting or taking laxatives. What is eaten and drunk should also be recorded. A measure of control is thus established and the basis for weekly discussion is provided. A group is a useful adjunct to keep the patient's interest and conscience alert.

REFERENCES

Asher, R. (1949) 'Myxoedematous Madness', *British Medical Journal, 2,* 555-62

Ballinger, C.B. (1976) 'Psychiatric Morbidity and the Menopause: Clinical Features', *British Medical Journal, 1,* 1183-5

Ballinger, C.B.W. A.(1985) 'The Menopause and the Climacteric', from Priest, R.G. (Ed.) *Psychological Disorders in Obstetrics and Gynaecology,* Butterworths, London and Boston

Beumont, P.J.V. (1979) Chapter 6 in Granville-Grossman, K. (Ed.) *Recent Advances in Clinical Psychiatry,* Churchill-Livingstone, London and New York

Bleuler, M. (1954) *Endokrinologische Psychiatrie,* Thieme, Stuttgart

Cropper, C.F.J. (1973) 'Hypothyroidism in Psychogeriatric Patients: Ankle-jerk Reaction as a Screening Test', *Gerontologia Clinica, 13,* 15-24

Dally, P. and Gomez, J. (1979) *Anorexia Nervosa,* Heinemann, London

Donovan, B.T. (1985) *Hormones and Human Behaviour,* Cambridge University Press, Cambridge

Dunbar, H.F. (1954) *Emotions and Bodily Change,* Columbia University Press, New York

Ford, C.V., Bray, G.A. and Swerdloff, R.S. (1976) 'A Psychiatric Study of Patients Referred with a Diagnosis of Hypoglycemia', *American Journal of Psychiatry, 133,* 290-4

Gibbons, J.L. (1983) Chapter 3 in Lader, M.H. (Ed.) *Mental Disorders and Somatic Illness,* Cambridge University Press, Cambridge

Gomez, J. and Scott, G. (1980) 'Hypothyroidism, Psychotropic Drugs and Cardiotoxicity', *British Journal of Psychiatry, 136,* 89-91

Hall, R.C.W. Popkin, M.K. Stickney, S.K. and Gardner, E. (1979) 'Presentation of the Steroid Psychoses', *Journal of Nervous and Mental Disease, 167,* 229-36

Henschke, P.T. and Pain, R.W. (1977) 'Thyroid Disease in a Psychogeriatric Population', *Age and Ageing, 6,* 151-5

Lishman, W. A. (1978) *Organic Psychiatry,* Blackwell, London

Marks, V. (1966) 'Spontaneous Hypoglycaemia', *Hospital Medicine, i*, 118-25

Marks, V.M. (1975) 'Hypoglycaemia II: Other Causes', *Clinics in Endocrinology and Metabolism, 5*, 769-82

Money, J. and Pollitt, E. (1966) 'Studies in the Psychology of Dwarfism', *Journal of Pediatrics, 68*, 381-91

Popkin, M.K. and Mackenzie, T.B. (1980) Chapter 9 in Hall R.C.W. (Ed.) Psychiatric Presentations of Somatic Illness, Spectrum, New York

Prange, A.J., Breese, G.R., Wilson, J.C. and Lipson, M.A. (1975) 'Pituitary and Supra-pituitary Hormones: Brain Behavioural Effects', in Sachar, E.J. (Ed.) *Topics in Psychoendocrinology*, Grune & Stratton, New York

Russell, G.F.M. (1979) 'Bulimia Nervosa: an Ominous Variant of Anorexia Nervosa', *Pyschological Medicine, 9*, 429-48

Sachar, E. (1975) 'Psychiatric Disturbances Associated with Endocrine Disorders', in Arieti, S. and Reiser, M. (Eds) *American Handbook of Psychiatry, 4*, Basic Books, New York

Turk, D.C. and Speers, M.A. (1983) 'Diabetes Mellitus: a Cognitive-Functional Analysis of Stress', in Burish, T.G. and Bradley, L.A. (Eds) *Coping with Chronic Disease*, Academic Press, New York

Webb, W.L. and Gehi, M. (1980) Chapter 16 in Hall, R.C.W. (Ed.) *Psychiatric Presentations of Somatic Illness*, Spectrum, New York

Whitlock, F.A. (1982) Chapter 7 in *Symptomatic Affective Disorders*, Academic Press, Sydney

Wolff, G. and Money, J. (1973) 'Relationship between Sleep and Growth in Patients with Reversible Somatrotropin Deficiency', *Psychological Mecicine, 3*, 18-27

10

Liaison in Renal and Genitourinary Problems

The genitourinary system subserves complex and diverse functions: excretion, homeostatic regulation of metabolism, blood pressure control, endocrine secretion, and sexual and reproductive activity. A selective review is made of the areas in which psychiatric liaison is most often required (Lukensmeyer, 1980).

URAEMIA

Cerebral pathology in uraemia is largely non-specific, depending on the underlying disease processes and secondary complications (Lishman, 1978). Impaired renal function is signalled by reduced creatinine clearance and by uraemia. Urea itself is non-toxic, but associated factors are an increase in brain permeability, reduced cerebral neutralisation of oxygen, varying electrolyte and acid-base values, hypertension, and disturbed neurotransmitter metabolism. Rapid changes are more likely to upset cerebral function than gradual. Secondary complications include anaemia, water intoxication, infection and thiamine deficiency.

Early symptoms associated with renal dysfunction may be regarded as depressive: apathy, fatigue, reduced concentration span, anorexia and sometimes headache (Wise, 1974). Or there may be an apparent personality deterioration with irritability, restlessness, insomnia and lack of thoughtfulness (Neary, 1976; Morgan, 1983). Any of these symptoms may arise in a medical patient and involve the liaisonist, emphasising the need to scrutinise laboratory results. Variations which may seem insignificant to physican colleagues may yet underlie psychological symptoms. Blood urea levels as low as 10 mmol/1 (normal range 3.2–6.6 mmol/l) are of interest. Causes of renal insufficiency to consider are kidney, prostate and bladder problems, ureteric back pressure from any cause, analgesic excess, dehydration, bleeding from the gut, shock, and age-related deterioration. It is towards these areas that the physician's attention should be directed.

Uraemic encephalopathy

Later manifestations also likely to concern the psychiatrist are slow, slurred speech; impaired memory; reduction in all activity including sexual; and episodes of disorientation, leading on to frank delirium and coma. Mental and neurological symptoms march together, with muscle twitching, tremor, rigidity, choreoathetosis, fits, proximal myopathy and peripheral neuropathy with burning feet and restless legs. Manic, paranoid, depressive or anxiety symptoms may precede an obvious acute organic brain syndrome.

Restoration of physiological normality is essential treatment with the avoidance as far as practicable of psychotropic medication, particularly sedatives. Because of increased brain permeability and reduced urinary excretion, toxic effects even of antibiotics are likely. Too rapid change towards normal may also make the mental symptoms worse temporarily. Psychiatric management comprises nursing in a well-lit open ward with plentiful reassurance and reminders of reality.

END STAGE RENAL DISEASE (ESRD)

Patients and their relatives and the staff who work in renal units are subject to intense emotional strains and conflicts. Those with ESRD have to contend with the physiological results of their disease, often affecting their psychological state directly as well as secondarily, for instance through impotence. Medication, especially hypotensives, may in itself be depressant; and these patients are in a desperate life situation. All are on borrowed time: they would be dead without treatment, whether haemodialysis, peritoneal dialysis or transplant.

A range of coping mechanisms may be called into play. Denial is the commonest, and although it helps the patient through unpleasant procedures, it may lead to non-compliance with treatment and emotional isolation, since he dare not risk being faced with reality. Displacement transfers feelings of anger about the disease on to relatives, staff and other fit people. Regression makes for convenient compliance at first but continues into the dependence and demandingness appropriate only to infancy. In the struggle for a sense of control the patient may become intolerably domineering and dictatorial (Czaczkes and Kaplan De Nour, 1978). Feelings to foster are realistic determination and motivation. Helplessness undermines this, so the patient needs to feel that he is still choosing what to do with his life, that there is more to it than the illness, and that he has personal worth. Each treatment modality carries its own problems.

Chronic hospital haemodialysis

The patient who receives his haemodialysis at hospital exchanges ultimately terminal illness for dependence on a machine, with curtailment of freedom geographically and in the choice of what to eat and drink and how much. Staff and patient expectations are likely to diverge: the latter tending to cleave to the familiar sick role and deferred responsibility, whereas the former are eager to stress improvement and how much more the patient can do. Yet if the patient takes the initiative in demonstrating his near-normality, the staff may react against this also. The pressures of dialysis life may outweigh the fear of death, and in some units withdrawal from treatment is made an explicit option (Dottes, 1980).

Renal unit staff also have an ambiguous role with technical apparatus as impressive as in an intensive therapy unit, but tending the same patients month after month in a drama played out slowly with some deaths but no lives fully restored. To encourage both independence and compliance is to walk a tightrope, leading to irritation and possessiveness.

The families of hospital dialysis patients have a fragmented life and the patient's assignments with his machine may seem like those with a mistress. Lack of sexual fulfilment and constraint upon planning family meals and holidays and financial uncertainty are additional burdens. Training a spouse later to help with home dialysis, blood and needles is far outside normal marital expectations (Pritchard, 1982).

Home haemodialysis

In general this increases the impact of the illness on the family while reducing inconvenience for the patient. A skilled and tactful home haemodialysis nurse provides training, reassurance and support to all parties. Nevertheless marital breakdown is not uncommon as a

167

result of rejection of a machine-ridden partnership.

Continuous ambulatory peritoneal dialysis (CAPD)

This is less problematical for the family but the patient himself is often constantly worried about the technique and finds it takes much of his time to manage. For women in particular there is an uncomfortable awareness of the distended abdomen, concern lest the catheter leaks, and constant anxiety that through a slip in hygiene peritonitis may develop. It is a possible method for those who live alone. The one haunting fear of CAPD patients, that the method reduces the chances of a successful transplant later, has recently been shown to be groundless (Donnelly *et al.*, 1985; Evangelista *et al.*, 1985).

Dysequilibrium syndrome

This short-lived but dramatic disorder may occur during or after haemodialysis, especially if there were severe metabolic abnormalities initially and dialysis has been rapid. A disparity of urea and other chemical levels between cerebrospinal fluid and plasma may be causative, or there may be reactive hypoglycaemia from the sugar in the dialysand, or hyponatraemia. It is an organic reaction but presents with symptoms that may be suspected of psychogenicity: restlessness, headache, nausea, disorientation, tremor, *grand mal* fits and hypertension. Psychological intervention is irrelevant, and treatment comprises the use of osmotically active solutes, shortening the periods on dialysis, reducing the blood-flow rate, and perhaps prophylactic anticonvulsants.

Dialysis encephalopathy: dementia dialytica

Wernicke's encephalopathy has been reported in dialysis patients on a restricted diet. More frequently a progressive organic brain syndrome specific to dialysis patients occurs, dialysis encephalopathy. It was first described by Alfrey *et al.* (1976). It is characterised by speech disorder, grimacing, tremor and myoclonus, with memory impairment, difficulty in concentration and conceptualisation. A rapidly deteriorating course usually ends in death in six to 12 months. Psychiatric advice is sometimes sought among other unsuccessful approaches. It appears that the cause is aluminium toxicity through accumulation from the water used in dialysis (MacDermott *et al.*, 1978). The most useful treatment is to stop giving aluminium hydroxide by mouth, and to reduce the aluminium in the dialysing fluid (Platts and Hislop, 1976).

Depression and suicide

Organicity can produce any kind of psychiatric disturbance and in its milder forms makes the patient less emotionally stable. It must be sought meticulously, together with laboratory investigations in renal patients. Nevertheless, because of their universality, the emotional reactions to ESRD and its treatment are of the greatest importance in liaison work. These have been touched upon briefly (see above), and competently reviewed by Salmons (1980). Anxiety and depression of clinical dimensions are found in 53 per cent of dialysis patients (Kaplan De Nour and Czaczkes, 1976). Farmer *et al.* (1979) detected 31 per cent of depressed patients in their dialysis sample, 27 per cent harbouring suicidal ideas. Antidepressant medication or — if necessary because of suicidal risk — ECT is effective. Gomez in an unpublished study presented in 1980 found a suicide rate of 195/100 000 among dialysis patients in England and, compared with 8/100 000 in the general population or 12.9/100 000 in those aged 35-64. If those who chose to die by refusing treatment are included, the suicide rate for dialysis patients increases to 456/100 000. Clearly this is a substantial risk, underlining the need for psychiatric support in renal units either directly with the patients or through guidance and support of the unit staff.

Renal transplantation

Although this, if it is successful, is the best ultimate answer to ESRD, it is shot through with potential problems. The necessary temporary routine isolation of the patient in the early postoperative period enhances natural anxiety by reducing sensory input and personal support. Immunosuppressant and steroid medication may increase any tendency to an organic reaction of confusion or even frank delirium, and, more seriously, leave the patient vulnerable to such infections, as meningoencephalitis, or to reticulo-endothelial tumour, especially involving the central nervous system.

Even without such mischances, the transplant patient is naturally anxious about the risk of rejection and a return to dialysis and sub-health. He also has doubts about the donor, if dead, or feels beholden to and concern for the donor if a relative. He often experiences a mix of guilt, gratitude and resentment. The relative who has made considerable, irrevocable, personal sacrifice will be particularly distressed by the possibility of rejection. These feelings may project on to the patient, producing a state of hostile interdependency. It is essential in considering relative-donor transplantation to exclude any with ambivalent feelings towards the patient or those so much subject to family coercion that freedom of choice is impaired.

Support for the transplant patient, his family including children, and for the donor and his marital partner where applicable is essential, on an individual and family basis. Group therapy for transplant patients as for those with malignant disease is fraught with the danger of demoralising disaster to one or another member underscoring the patient's helplessness rather than promoting healthy, positive responses (Eisendrath, 1976).

BENIGN PROSTATIC HYPERTROPHY

Usually the symptoms of age-related prostatic enlargement are urinary, and recognised for what they are even by the patient: nocturia, daytime frequency, hesitancy, urgency and dribbling, in variable degrees. However, the constitutional symptoms of fatigue and flank pain may be prominent, and the problems misinterpreted as of psychological origin. A more unfortunate occasional presentation is marked and unexpected sexual excitement from pelvic vasocongestion. Psychiatric advice may be requested when — say — an elderly bishop is accused of indecent behaviour.

If obstruction develops slowly, the first presentation may be with uraemia: manifest in pseudo-depression or psycho-organic symptoms as described earlier. Since prostatic hypertrophy is a disorder of elderly men, other debilitating disease or intellectual deterioration may cloud the issue and the patient may not be competent to give a fully revealing history. Sudden urinary obstruction with or without infection may arise spontaneously or in reaction to anticholinergic effects with for instance, tricyclic antidepressants, neuroleptics or anti-parkinsonian medication. An acute organic brain syndrome may result in a patient with previously undiagnosed prostatic disease. Postoperative delirium is not uncommon in patients undergoing prostatic procedures, and should be dealt with as described in Chapter 3.

Adult enuresis

Recurrent involuntary voiding of urine usually arises in childhood and may be primary or secondary. Apart from rare organic causes it is associated with developmental delay, habit deficiency and/or profound insecurity. In 85 per cent it occurs only at night, usually but not invariably in the first period of stage 4 sleep. In 1 per cent the problem continues into adulthood and comes to notice when the patient is hospitalised, joins the Services or marries. Early childhood insecurity has become chronic anxiety, often dealt with by the patient by heavy drinking. This worsens but 'excuses' the situation. As with enuretic children, behavioural methods including an alarm and a reward system, and tricyclic antidepressant treatment should be applied: for example imipramine 75 mg at night. Occasionally the REM-suppressant action of phenelzine is more successful: doses of 45-90 mg daily are desirable if well-tolerated. In adults simultaneous psychotherapy is also necessary, including the wife if any, since she is likely to be unintentionally maintaining the habit. Patients who first develop enuresis in adult life and in whom there is no local pathology, nor, for instance, evidence of multiple sclerosis, are likely to be acutely psychiatrically ill. Hysterical regression, acute schizophrenia, delusional depression or the frontal lobe syndrome should be considered during the diagnostic mental state evaluation. The elderly demented person may become incontinent; more often a urinary infection arises in an old person, and appropriate treatment and help in re-establishing a good habit removes the problem.

LIAISON IN SEXUAL DISORDERS

Psychosomatic disorders

The numbers attending clinics for sexually transmitted diseases (STD) have increased five-fold over the last quarter century. During that time the proportion of women has risen from one in 14 to one in two. Over 70 per cent of patients turn out not to have any form of STD. Some have understandable worries, or are projecting sexual or other emotional problems on to the genital organs. Some have experienced attacks of venereal disease previously, and many complain of symptoms which are consistent with a physical disorder.

Persistent vulval irritation is frequently attributed to thrush by younger women, but when there is no infection is likely to be symptomatic of fear — whether or not justifiable — of losing their sexual partner. In older women atrophic vaginitis may coexist and cloud the issue, but the intensity of the symptom is disproportionate to the local disorder. A feeling of sexual deprivation can be elicited gently in some cases, and discussion is a relief. Persistent vulval, perineal, perianal or vaginal burning or pain is particularly intractable in those of obsessional personality. This type is also vulnerable to tension and depression, and an empirical trial of psychotropic medication, particularly an MAOI, may be worthwhile. The physical symptoms are likely to defeat all apparently appropriate treatment and come to provide a major focus in the patient's life, albeit distressing.

Reported vaginal discharge which cannot be demonstrated by examination or pathological tests may result from any of a range of sexual anxieties and inadequacy. An authoritative, correct, functional diagnosis cuts short a complaint that is readily perpetuated by the doctor's expression of doubt. 'Phantom thrush' is a synonym for dyspareunia of psychological origin, frequently based on a genuine candidal attack long since cured. Slightly more women than men develop psychosomatic problems, but men who are anxious or depressed may have symptoms characteristic of non-specific urethritis, such as frequency, dysuria, perineal discomfort and testicular aching.

Venereophobia

There is a steady flow of patients to clinics for genitourinary disorders who are afraid they have contracted venereal disease. Their numbers have escalated in the last four years, first from the media attention accorded to herpes genitalis, and then — dramatically — with the advent of AIDS (acquired immune deficiency syndrome). Some patients run substantial risks, for instance call girls, homosexual men and the inveterately promiscuous. Most are reassured by careful physical examination and appropriate microbiological and serological tests. For others such procedures do nothing to relieve their anxieties. They return repeatedly, aiming to see a different doctor each time, and do the rounds of the clinics and private practitioners.

The disease which such patients used to dread was syphilis, but nowadays syphilophobia affects only the over-fifties. Gonorrhoea and NSU (non-specific urethritis) were major preoccupations among this type of patient in the 1970s, by whom the slightest normal moisture was reported as evidence of urethral discharge. Herpetiphobia reached a peak in 1984 (Oates and Gomez, 1984). Nowadays it is so completely overshadowed by AIDS panic that a woman who had been raped in particularly unpleasant circumstances was scarcely worried at all when she found she had acquired herpes, so long as she did not have AIDS. Anything to do with sexual activity is spangled with guilt, and an unjustified conviction of having VD is likely to be symptomatic of a more fundamental psychological disorder, and is merely the vehicle for fear or self-depreciation, much as with cancerphobia (Chapter 13). Anxiety states, depression (either neurotic or psychotic and even delusional) or hypochondriasis serving hysterical avoidance mechanisms, may present as venereophobia. Women in particular may use physical symptoms as an escape from sexual activity. Treatment is of the underlying disorder.

Herpes genitalis

Anxiety and reactive depression may be understandable responses to herpes, particularly since this is a relapsing condition with a potential for infecting others including the newborn and has an association with cancer in women. As with herpes labialis, emotional upset may precipitate an attack: fortunately a course of acyclovir taken from just before and during a holiday ensures freedom of recurrence in the particular chosen period. Continued, crippling anxiety over herpes is usually causally related to problems with the sexual partner in particular, and requires exploration. Serious sexual difficulties may result if a partner has or is suspected of having herpes. Psychotherapy and medication may be required, and specific sexual guidance in the latter cases.

AIDS

Those who are asymptomatic but serologically positive for the HIV virus require support. Their situation is frightening, isolating and often involves regrets. Self-help groups do extremely valuable work, and therapist-led groups and individual counselling and psychotherapy are available but are used less than anticipated. Clinical anxiety states and depression may be precipitated and call for specific treatment. For those in whom the disease develops, for instance with Kaposi's

173

sarcoma in obvious areas, social, occupational and personal rejection is inevitable and often devastating even if the response to treatment is favourable. AIDS encephalopathy should be remembered as a possibility in seropositive cases and manifests like other organic brain syndromes. With current prognostications a vast increase in psychiatric back-up for genitourinary diseases clinics is going to be required. Depression in seropositive patients frequently manifests in bowel symptoms and weight loss, which may be interpreted as evidence of advancing viral disease.

SEXUAL DYSFUNCTION

Sexual problems often come to light in the context of other medical disorders which may be considered to play a causative role. In fact in only 15-20 per cent of reported cases is there a significant organic component and this is probably an overestimate (Crown and d'Ardenne, 1982). It has been assessed that among educated, middle-class 'normal' married couples, 50 per cent of the men and 77 per cent of the women feel that they have sexual difficulties. Perception of such difficulties depends upon the affective tone of the association (Frank *et al.*, 1978). Sexual problems extend in a continuum from doubts, dissatisfaction and dysfunctions to definite disabilities. They include low libido in either sex; in men erectile and ejaculatory problems and penile pain; in women vaginismus, dyspareunia, anorgasmia and vulval burning. Psychogenicity is by far the commonest aetiological factor but organicity must be considered if only to exclude it. In women gynaecological disorders such as endometriosis and pelvic inflammatory disease cannot be forgotten, and in men prostatic disorders. In both sexes, but more obviously important in the male, relevant disorders are: trauma to the genitalia, pelvic bones or spinal cord; postoperative complications from rectal, bladder, uterine or prostatic surgery; chronic and debilitating disease and specific medical conditions, e.g. diabetes mellitus, ESRD, multiple sclerosis, and neuropathies. Drugs which may interfere with either erection or ejaculation include hypotensives, neuroleptics, anticholinergics, antidepressants — either tricyclic or MAOI, cytotoxics, oestrogens, alcohol and illicit social drugs. It is worth noting that diabetes has an exaggerated reputation as a specific cause of impotence. Lester *et al.* (1980) found 23 per cent of diabetic men to be impotent compared with 20 per cent of other medical outpatients. Nevertheless a minimal laboratory screen should include blood glucose, thyroxine level and liver function tests.

Investigation for psychogenic factors, in the context of a full history, should focus on sociocultural, educational and cognitive aspects; interpersonal relationship difficulties, especially power struggles; and intrapsychic conflicts, such as anxiety, anger and guilt (Gendel and Bonner, 1984). Loss of libido is symptomatic of a depressive state, and if this is of clinical proportions will recover with standard antidepressant therapies, chemical, cognitive or other.

Where it is assessed that the psychological aspects are largely responsible for sexual dysfunction, treatment is nearly always ineffective unless both partners are seen and are involved. Warmth, sympathy and encouragement are needed in liberal quantities, embedded in limitless patience on the part of the therapist whatever type of treatment is given. The patients suffer by turns from feelings of anxiety, humiliation, guilt and resentment, with all-pervading self-doubt which destroys sexual ease. The Masters and Johnston (1970) techniques of removing — temporarily — the challenge of having to perform full intercourse and concentrating initially on sensate focusing is a helpful approach in most cases, with stop-and-start or squeeze manoeuvre for premature ejaculation. Relaxation therapy is effective, sometimes in conjunction with graduated dilators, in vaginismus and female dyspareunia. Intractable vulval, perianal or penile soreness or burning not due to visible, obvious, local disorder is often associated with depression and upset or angry feelings towards the opposite sex, whether or not the current partner. Treatment by discussion and relaxation techniques is usually successful only in conjunction with MAOI treatment for at least two months for example phenelzine 30-45 mg or tranylcypromine 10-30 mg daily, before 4 p.m. Sexual tension is more wearing and searing than any other. In cases of low sexual drive, if the Masters and Johnson approach is ineffective, Gillan's (1979) stimulation therapy may be applied. This is most suitable for the primary cases and younger rather than middle-aged patients. In general, short active intervention is more effective than long-term insight-oriented therapy in these cases (Kaplan, 1974).

As a final resort, in cases of erectile impotence who are highly motivated and retain psychological desire and a minimum of some sensation, surgical assistance with a penile prosthesis, inflatable or rigid, may be employed. A new penile injection has shown promising results.

Specific handicaps

A special group are those whose sexual difficulties result from mutilating surgery, ranging from breast lumpectomy or mastectomy, through ostomies to vulvectomy or penile amputation. Mechanical as well as psychological problems may be posed by arthritis, obesity, muscular weakness, amputation or paralyses. Although ingenious sexual aids are available and help some patients, it is often emotionally impossible for the partners of such patients to fulfil expectations of sexual intimacy. For this reason, if the patient's own sexual interest has declined, measures to reflate it should be avoided unless there is absolute certainty that both partners are keen to have full intercourse. It may be more practicable to help them to obtain maximal pleasure from the parasexual activities of kissing, cuddling and massage. In other cases where it is mainly a matter of restoring confidence and retraining lost sensations, the Masters and Johnson method may be modified for individual needs.

SEXUAL ASSAULT

Rape, which by definition involves vaginal penetration, and other forms of sexual violence have become more frequent. They have reached almost epidemic proportions in some parts of the USA and are catching up in the UK. They occur particularly in episodes of civil disorder when susceptible young men are carried away by feelings of power and excitement. Women and children of either sex are the victims, and it is only in the last decade that the damage that they suffer directly and in the longer term has been recognised (Mezey, 1985).

Rape victims urgently need physical examination for trauma and traces of semen, and tests for pregnancy and the various sexually transmissible diseases. They also need an immediate opportunity and strong encouragement to speak of their experience and their feelings and fears, then and now. Almost invariably both children and adults who have been assaulted sexually feel illogically guilty and ashamed, dirty and unfit to mix with other people. They find excuses not to tell their parents and other nearest and dearest. If the subject is not aired and discussed over and over, particularly with important other people, until it has lost its emotional power, it is likely to lead to clinical depression later, to phobias relating to the place and circumstances of the episode, and an intractable difficulty in forming normal relationships with men. Those who are politically committed to the concepts of female oppression and male aggression are only too ready to support rape victims, but what is even more valuable for rapid and complete psychological restoration is to receive help from men, and also from women without political bias. Parents, boyfriends and best friends need to be involved, but after three months in which free discussion is desirable, the victim should no longer be encouraged to talk about the incident. Similarly a childhood rape revealed years afterwards in adult life should not be made the subject of long, intense discussion. To reopen this type of wound, long if not perfectly healed, is counterproductive.

Child assault victims, like adults, need to be helped to talk about what happened, but without being engulfed by adult indignation on their behalf. If the molester was a family member, a few family group discussions including him and a professional are useful and reassuring to the child and the others. A shorter period for all the discussion is appropriate in cases involving children.

PROBLEMS ASSOCIATED WITH HOMOSEXUALITY

Female homosexuality seldom leads to liaison psychiatric involvement, although lesbians are rather more likely than the generality of women to drink heavily. Male homosexuals are again having to face social disapproval and rejection since the advent of AIDS. The fear of infection from past or present cottaging or other forms of promiscuity is sharpened. AIDS aside, harmful sadomasochistic practices and damage to the rectal mucosa, or worse, are specific dangers for the active male homosexual, which may bring him to hospital. Alcohol-related problems are also common in this group (Ziebold and Mongeon, 1982). These men are often sensitive and insecure and may lack family support, so that overdosage is far likelier than in others. They need especial understanding and reassurance when in medical difficulties, and may prefer to discuss personal problems with a psychiatrist rather than their surgeon or physician. A few ask for help in converting to heterosexuality, and if this is a genuine, sustained wish, referral to a unit specialising in behavioural methods for sexual problems is the best course.

REFERENCES

Alfrey, A.C., Le Gendre, G.R. and Kaehny, W.D. (1976) 'The Dialysis Encephalopathy Syndrome: Possible Aluminium Intoxication', *New England Journal of Medicine, 294*, 184-8

Crown, S. and d'Ardenne, P. (1982) Symposium on Sexual Dysfunction: 'Controversies, Methods, Results', *British Journal of Psychiatry, 140*, 70-7

Czaczkes, J.W. and Kaplan De Nour, A. (1978) *Chronic Haemodialysis as a Way of Life*, Brunner/Mazel, New York

Donnelly, P.K., Lennàrd, T.W.J., Proud, E., Taylor, R.M.R., Henderson, R., Fletcher, K., Elliot, W., Ward, M.K. and Wilkinson, R. (1985) 'Continuous Ambulatory Peritoneal Dialysis and Renal Transplantation', *British Medical Journal, 291*, 1000-3

Dottes, A.L. (1980) *Dialysis and Transplantation, 9*, 732-40

Eisendrath, R.M. (1976) 'Adaptations to Renal Transplantation', in Howells, J.G. (Ed.) *Modern Perspectives in the Psychiatric Aspects of Surgery*, Macmillan, London

Evangelista, J.B., Bennett-Jones, D., Cameron, J.S., Ogg, C., Williams, D.G., Taube, D.H., Neild, G. and Rudge, C. (1985) 'Renal Transplantation in Patients Treated with Haemodialysis and Short and Long Term Continuous Ambulatory Peritoneal Dialysis', *British Medical Journal, 291*, 1004-7

Farmer, C.J., Snowden, S.A. and Parsons, V. (1979) 'The Prevalence of Psychiatric Illness among Patients on Home Dialysis', *Psychological Medicine, 9*, 509-14

Frank, E., Anderson, C. and Rubinstein, D. (1978) 'Frequency of Sexual Dysfunction in "Normal" Couples', *New England Journal of Medicine, 299*, 111-15

Gendel, E.S. and Bonner, E.J. (1984) 'Psychosexual Dysfunction', in Goldman, H.H. (Ed.) *Review of General Psychiatry*, Lange, California

Gillan, P. (1979) 'Stimulation Therapy for Sexual Dysfunction', *British Journal of Sexual Medicine, 6, 13-14*

Kaplan, H.S. (1974) *The New Sex Therapy*, Brunner/Mazel, New York

Kaplan De Nour, A. and Czaczkes, J.W. (1976) 'The Influence of Personality on Adjustment to Chronic Dialysis', *Journal of Nervous and Mental Disease, 162*, 323-33

Lester, E., Grant, A.J. and Woodroffe, F.J. (1980) 'Impotence in Diabetic and Non-diabetic Hospital Out-patients', *British Medical Journal, 281*, 354-5

Lishman, W.A. (1978) Chapter II in *Organic Psychiatry*, Blackwell, London

Lukensmeyer, W.W. (1980) 'Psychiatric Presentations of Selected Genitourinary Disorders', in Hall, R.C.W. (Ed.) *Psychiatric Presentations of Medical Illness*, Spectrum, New York

MacDermott, J.R., Smith, A.I., Ward, M.K., Parkinson, I.S. and Kerr, D.N.S. (1978) 'Brain Aluminium Concentration in Dialysis Encephalopathy', *Lancet, 1*, 901-3

Masters, W.H. and Johnson, V.E. (1970) *Human Sexual Inadequacy*, Churchill, Edinburgh

Mezey, G.C. (1985) 'Rape — Victimological and Psychiatric Aspects',

British Journal of Hospital Medicine, 33, 152-58

Morgan, H.G. (1983) Chapter 2 in Lader, M.H. (Ed.) *Mental Disorders and Somatic Illness*, Cambridge University Press, Cambridge

Neary, D.C. (1976) 'Neuropsychiatric Sequelae of Renal Failure', *British Journal of Hospital Medicine, 15*, 122-30

Oates, J.K. and Gomez, J. (1984) 'Venereophobia', *British Journal of Hospital Medicine, 31*, 435-36

Platts, M.M. and Hislop, J.S. (1976) 'Aluminium and Dialysis Encephalopathy', *Lancet, 2*, 98

Pritchard, M. (1982) 'Psychological Pressure in a Renal Unit', *British Journal of Hospital Medicine, 27*, 512-17

Salmons, P.H. (1980) 'Psychosocial Aspects of Chronic Renal Failure', *British Journal of Hospital Medicine, 23*, 617-22

Wise, T.N. (1974) 'The Pitfalls of Diagnosing Depression in Chronic Renal Disease, *Psychosomatics, 15*, 83-4

Ziebold, T.O. and Mongeon, J.E. (Eds) (1982) *Alcoholism and Homosexuality,* Haworth Press, New York

11

Liaison in Bone and Joint Problems

The musculoskeletal system is the largest in the body and serves all activities involving movement, from heavy labour to microsurgery. A fractured bone causes immediate immobility at least of part of the body and more insidiously developing pain and stiffness are commonplace. Either type of disability may involve the psychiatrist.

BACKACHE

Back problems account for 2 per cent of all general practitioners' consultations and 25 per cent of orthopaedic referrals. Major spinal disasters are usually straightforward surgical matters, but *chronic low back pain* (CLBP) often has a multifactorial aetiology, sometimes predominantly psychosomatic. Psychiatric opinion is likely to be sought if there appears to be insufficient organic pathology to account for the symptoms, and they persist. Nevertheless it is wise to have in mind the range of possible causes of CLBP:

(a) *Traumatic and mechanical problems.* Most people suffer musculotendinous or ligament strain at some time, and fat middle-aged women with lumbar hyperlordosis are particularly liable to develop chronic lumbosacral strain (Waddell, 1982).

(b) *Degenerative changes.* Spondylosis affecting the intervertebral discs and osteoarthrosis of the facet joints are normal concomitants of ageing. The symptoms — oddly — are at their worst when the patient is in his or her 50s or 60s but produce less trouble later. A middle-aged patient can be reassured that backache at 50 does not mean crippledom at 70.

(c) *Inflammatory diseases.* Only two are of importance in liaison work: tuberculosis, usually in an immigrant, and ankylosing spondylitis in a young adult. Sacroiliitis and a high erythrocyte sedimentation rate characterise the latter.

(d) *Neoplasia*. Myelomatosis may cause back pain, or metastases from a primary in the lung, breast, thyroid, prostate,kidney or occasionally the colon.

(e) *Referred pain*. This may be visceral, for instance from a posterior duodenal ulcer; retroperitoneal, for instance from carcinoma of the pancreas; urinary; gynaecological; or pelvic, for instance from cancer of the rectum.

(f) *Emotionally mediated pain*. Depression or a chronic tension state may be the primary disorder underlying back symptoms (Edgar, 1984).

Since a large number of patients suffer chronic or recurrent backache which interferes with their pattern of living disproportionately to the degree of structural damage or abnormality, Garron and Leavitt (1983) have constructed a Back Pain Classification Scale aimed at identifying those whose symptoms derive from psychological disorder. They have employed the Minnesota Multiphasic Personality Inventory (MMPI), the State-Trait Anxiety Scale and the Social Readjustment Rating Scale to build their scale. McGill *et al*. in the same year (1983) found that patients with chronic low back pain scored highly on the hypochondriasis profile in the MMPI, but that the results were of no predictive value.

More recently Schmidt (1985) found that CLBP patients with a negative self-concept, feelings of inadequacy and a rigid, mistrustful temperament do particularly badly. These features are not dependent on the duration of the disorder. Such patients are likely to feel subjectively exhausted after minor effort, and fail to persist with exercise and physiotherapeutic treatment. Their verbal and performance behaviours indicating pain are often sustained by the positive reinforcement of sympathy, medication and relief from irksome responsibilities. Along similar lines Slade and his colleagues (1983) examined 91 students who had previously suffered back pain, from a sample of 165. A poor prognosis was associated with passive coping responses, i.e. rest and withdrawal, whereas a confrontational style, carrying on regardless of pain, seemed to lead to a better long-term outcome with fewer relapses. A fear-avoidance mechanism was thought to induce exaggerated pain perception.

Management of CLBP must include medication for any depression or tension and discussion of personal problems and conflicts, where relevant. This is usually the case, whether the psychiatric condition is primary or secondary. Operant conditioning and cognitive-behavioural manoeuvres are also necessary by the time the backache has become well established (see Chapter 16). Maladaptive patterns of thought and behavour will have developed.

GENERAL MUSCULOSKELETAL PAINS

Harvey Moldofsky (1976) describes what Galen, Sydenham and others had already observed: a syndrome of widespread aching and stiffness, chronic fatigue, impaired work performance, poor sleep and emotional distress. Various terms have been applied: neurasthenia, myalgia, psychogenic rheumatism and fibrositis syndrome. None is apt, although the cluster of symptoms is well recognised and prevalent. Moldofsky's hypothesis, based on two small studies, is that the key factor is lack of stage 4 sleep associated with morning stiffness, muscular tenderness and aching, heaviness, low miserable mood and tiredness in those leading predominantly sedentary lives. They are often middle-aged and middle-class. In his patient sample all had experienced an upsetting event or stressful domestic situation at the onset of the sleep disturbance and other symptoms. Once started, a cycle of muscle tension, pain, fatigue and irritiability is self-perpetuating. Management may be in the hands of generalist, rheumatologist or psychiatrist and involves exploration of ways of coping with the patient's particular conflict or anxiety-provoking factors; regular exercise, started in the physiotherapy department; and restoration of a normal sleep pattern without the use of hypnotics or alcohol, which reduce stage 4 sleep. A hot drink at bedtime and relaxation or autohypnotic techniques should follow a sufficiently active day.

Chronic neck and shoulder pain

This is a somewhat similar condition with concomitant depression of mood and failure to cope with normal commitments, such as shopping, cooking or office routine. Grosshandler (1985) suggests a mixed aetiology and management directed towards an adjustment in which pain is no longer the dominant factor in the patient's life. A multidisciplinary approach is useful in all chronic musculoskeletal disorders.

Non-steroidal anti-inflammatory medication is helpful temporarily but the side-effects may be damaging (see Chapter 15). Chronic use of minor analgesics is also undesirable, but antidepressants are useful both for their mood-elevating and their analgesic effects. A trigger point injection can give a good start to psychotherapeutic treatment, and hypnoanalgesia is often successful. It is counterproductive to offer indefinite support and help, and the duration of a course of treatment should be set in advance.

RHEUMATOID ARTHRITIS

This disease involves gross physical symptoms buts its aetiology has long been a battleground between those hypothesising a particular personality type and response pattern as overwhelmingly important and those concentrating on hereditary and constitutional factors, who regard the depression often seen in rheumatoid arthritis as an understandable reaction to the disease.

Nearly 50 per cent of patients with rheumatoid arthritis, particularly women, are clinically depressed. Rimon, Dudley Hart and others, quoted by Whitlock (1982), find antidepressants helpful both for the psychiatric symptoms and for pain. The latter may be due to the mild analgesic effects of tricyclic drugs. Cerebral involvement is reliably documented but rare in rheumatoid arthritis and unlikely to be the cause of the depression so commonly encountered. However, both non-steroidal anti-inflammatory and steroid medication used in the disorder may contribute to depression (see Chapter 15). The interplay between emotional and organic factors is complex. A recent study of 74 women with rheumatoid arthritis demonstrated a clear division into two groups. One, termed the major conflict group, showed a correlation between the disease and distressing life events; the other group showed predominant hereditary influences (Rimon and Laakso, 1985). A sudden onset of the symptoms is likely to be related to an important psychogenic input, but asynchrony between mood and joint symptoms is of poor prognosis (Morgan, 1983). The personality type most likely to respond psychosomatically to emotional upset is duty-oriented, self-sacrificing and denying of resentments and hostility. Such people appear both timid and angry, with neither feeling acknowledged.

Daughters whose potential for happiness and fulfilment is distorted by 'having to' care for a domineering relative are in the risk group. Nevertheless, it seems that it is when the patient is relased from her responsibilities that the symptoms of rheumatoid arthritis emerge.

Similarly, a wife who was tied by her sense of propriety to an alcoholic waster at last decided to leave him: within a fortnight she was stricken down with severe joint symptoms. She had to return, and during the five years since then has never become sufficiently mobile to go out alone.

Medical and psychosocial support is needed by rheumatoid patients, with antidepressant medication in some (see above).

WRITERS' CRAMP

Views on this disorder illustrate the divergence between psychiatrists and other physicians about musculoskeletal symptoms. Writers' cramp affects most disastrously pianists and typists. It comprises spasm of the palm of the writing hand in particular, spreading to involve the arm and shoulder. It is naturally enhanced by anxiety, and in the early stages of the disorder the patient often finds that alcohol brings relief and the doctor prescribes diazepam with some benefit. MAOIs are dramatically helpful in some tense, perfectionist patients; phenelzine 30-60 mg or tranylcypromine 20-40 mg daily, before 4 pm. Others are helped by relaxation training. However, subtle indications of involvement of the basal ganglia may develop and it is probable that many cases in which writers' cramp is an isolated symptom are organic in origin.

Sheehy and Marsden (1982) found no increased prevalence of psychiatric morbidity in patients with writers' cramp using the Present State Examination. On the other hand Reger and his colleagues (1981) studied one case in depth with computerised tomography, regional blood-flow studies in the brain and dopamine betahydroxy-lase estimations after levodopa loading. The results were normal and psychological treatment led to marked improvement.

Linton and Gotestam's study (1985) demonstrating a moderate correlation between anxiety and muscle tension, is relevant to most of the disorders discussed.

SPORTS INJURIES

Health consciousness has become an obsession in the West, with diet as one facet, exercise another. Professional sport provides many present-day heroes and millionaires. Although sportsmen and women have become ever more skilful, the proportion who are injured is also increasing. Sports injuries fall into three groups:

1. undoubted injury with appropriate symptoms;
2. pain without significant apparent injury;
3. faking.

It is important to predict particular vulnerability to injury and prevent undue risk-taking. Many of the relevant factors are psychosocial, for instance family instability. A young competitor who has lost a parent runs five times the normal likelihood of injury (Yaffe, 1983). Life events, particularly losses and exits, increase the risk of impaired judgement to the point of recklessness, and those with a high self-concept are apt to take chances as they cannot easily conceive of failure. An exaggerated desire to demonstrate masculinity, or to show that women are as good as men, drives others towards injury.

Intense competitiveness in sport today can produce anxiety, to which a counterphobic response is to be even more daring. Some sportsmen have unrealistically stringent aims and indulge in an excess of high risk-taking; they almost welcome injury to atone for the slightest failure. Others, impelled by parental rather than their own ambition to take part in competitive sport, also meet injury half way: to punish their parents and provide an escape.

The dread of failure, far worse than physical fear, may lead a patient into injury-provoking behaviour, or to making much of a minor injury, or even pretending disability, to avoid competing. Truly psychosomatic mechanisms may operate also, and an emotional problem is somatised. The meaning to the patient of the injury must be elicited: this is usually a time-consuming process. Treatment can then begin.

Self-induced injury

It is not surprising that competitors sometimes fail to report an injury or symptoms of strain for fear of being forbidden to practise at a critical time. They may take analgesics, try to ignore the pain or dissociate from it, or attempt to persuade a doctor to give them cortisone or analgesic injections while increasing the damage by unremitting overuse.

Morgan, quoted by Yaffe (1983), described what he called a negative addiction to sport such as jogging. The daily run becomes overwhelmingly preoccupying, more important than wife, work or strained muscles and ligaments. Deprived of his regular dosage of exercise the patient becomes irritable, depressed and restless, requiring anxiolytics and psychotherapy to help towards adjustment to a more reasonable regimen. The effect of exercise in increasing endorphin levels is likely to be an aetiological factor in the seeming addiction and withdrawal symptoms.

Psychological consequences of sports injury

In general, injured sportsmen require different management according to their personality type. Introverts require reassurance and encouragement to return to their previous activity. Extraverts need holding back until they are physically recovered or they will undo the good achieved by rest and treatment by their enthusiasm.

Disability can be something akin to bereavement and is especially demoralising to the ageing male athlete. he may respond with hypochondriasis and panic attacks.

Treatment and prophylaxis

In sports psychiatry, treatment and prophylaxis may cover similar ground. It is noteworthy that 14 per cent of the 418 medical complaints made by the British Olympic Team in Moscow in 1984 were emotionally mediated stress reactions. Such techniques as relaxation, physical and psychological; cognitive skills training; positive thinking and mental rehearsal are all helpful (see Chapter 16). Attention-control practice helps to focus concentration on the task in hand, and biofeedback may be used to modify autonomic responses. More personally directed psychotherapy also has an important place for the individual under strain.

Signals

Signals indicating rising tension before a competition include:

1. a chance in arousal, reflected in marked increase or decrease in activity:
2. increased muscle tension especially in the neck and jaw;

3. facial muscular twitching;
4. hyperventilation;
5. yawning, stretching, coughing (common tension-reducing responses).

In such a situation of tension, injury is more likely, but may be ameliorated or averted. The first necessity is to get into eye contact, physical contact and verbal contact with the patient. Reassure him or her that his feelings of tension and his responses are normal in the circumstances. Distract him from direct contemplation of the ordeal to come by peripheral observations; and encourage some such mild physical activity as running on the spot to relax his muscles.

ACCIDENTS

Accidents are often not what they seem and psychological understanding and management may be vital.

> *Case 1*: A public relations officer of 48 fell from her fifth-floor balcony apparently by accident. In fact she had swallowed 100 diazepam tablets while balanced on the balustrade, and fell when she became unconscious. She was so relaxed that despite several fractures she survived. She was severely depressed but had consulted no one.
>
> *Case 2*: A girl of 19 holidaying abroad climbed a tree and fell, breaking her back. She had developed a manic illness, precipitated by marihuana, and believed she was meeting an extraterrestrial halfway to the sky.

Others who may have accidents, especially involving vehicles, are those who abuse hallucinogens or alcohol; schizophrenics who may behave bizarrely in the middle of a busy road; and patients who wander because of chronic organic brain disease. A catastrophic reaction may cause even the undemented elderly to freeze or dither in the path of oncoming disaster on wheels. Sometimes those urgently trying to escape from the police run into other dangers and sustain injuries. Injuries and mental suffering due to accidents which involve compensation deserve particularly careful assessment. Slowness of recovery often marches with the painful slowness of the legal machine. Malingering is rare in such cases, but unconscious mechanisms may well maintain the symptoms until a settlement is reached.

Accident proneness

Drink, drugs and physical disability are all potent factors. Personal difficulties and a plethora of life events may impair concentration (Connolly, 1981). Psychiatric disorders such as schizophrenia, depression, anxiety state or mania impair judgement, as do organic states such as epilepsy, dementia, frontal lobe lesions and some sequelae of head injury. Women are said to be more accident prone in the paramenstruum.

Children may also be accident prone, due to the mild clumsiness of minimal brain damage; hyperactivity; undiagnosed deafness or defective vision. In cases of recurrent 'accidents', the possibility of non-accidental injury should be considered. There is usually conflict or deprivation in the parental background (see Chapter 8).

REFERENCES

Connolly, J. (1981) 'Accident Proneness', *British Journal of Hospital Medicine, 26,* 470-81

Edgar, M.A. (1984) 'Backache', *British Journal of Hospital Medicine, 32,* 290-301

Garron, D.C. and Leavitt, F. (1983) 'Psychological and Social Correlates of the Back Pain Classification Scale', *Journal of Personality Assessment, 47,* 60-5

Grosshandler, S.L., Strates, N.E., Toomey, T.C. and Gray, W.F. (1985) 'Chronic Neck and Shoulder Pain', *Postgraduate Medicine, 77,* 149-59

Linton, S.J. and Gotestam, K.G. (1985) 'Relations between Pain, Anxiety, Mood and Muscle Tension in Chronic Pain Patients', *Psychotherapy and Psychosomatics, 43,* 90-5

McGill, J.C., Lawlis, G.F. and Selby, D. (1983) 'The Relationship of the Minnesota Multiphasic Personality Inventory Profile Clusters to Pain Behaviours', *Journal of Behavioural Medicine, 6,* 77-92

Moldofsky, H. (1976) 'Psychogenic Rheumatism or the Fibrositis Syndrome', in Hill, O. (Ed.) *Modern Trends in Psychosomatic Medicine — 3,* Butterworths, London

Morgan, H. (1983) 'General Medical Disorders', in Lader, M.H. (Ed.) *Mental Disorders and Somatic Illness,* Cambridge University Press, Cambridge

Reger, I., Vardi, I., Bornstein, N. and Shapira, T. (1981) 'Writers' Cramp: Psychological Aspects', *Harefuah, 100,* 523-5, and 550

Rimon, R. and Laakso, R.L. (1985) 'Life Stress and Rheumatoid Arthritis: a 15-year Follow-up Study', *Psychotherapy and Psychosomatics, 43,* 38-43

Schmidt, A.J.M. (1985) 'Cognitive Factors in the Performance Level of

Chronic Low Back Pain Patients', *Journal of Psychosomatic Research, 29,* 183-9

Sheehy, M.P. and Marsden, C.D. (1982) 'Writers' Cramp: a Focal Dystonia', *Brain and Journal of Neurology, 105,* 461-80

Slade, P.D., Tromp, J.D.G., Letham, J. and Bentley, G. (1983) 'The Fear-avoidance Model of Exaggerated Pain Perception', *Behavioural Research and Therapy, 21,* 409-13

Waddell, G. (1982) 'An Approach to Backache', *British Journal of Hospital Medicine, 28,* 187-219

Whitlock, F.A. (1982) 'Immunological Diseases', from *Symptomatic Affective Disorders,* Academic Press, Sydney

Yaffe, M. (1983) 'Sports Injuries: Psychological Aspects', *British Journal of Hospital Medicine, 29,* 224-32

12

Liaison in Dermatology and Infections

Skin and nervous tissue derive from the same embryonic layer, and disturbances in either system affect the other. The most primitive and emotive sensory modality is mediated through the skin, and emotions are reflected in cutaneous change, for example the blush of shame or the piloerection of fear. Medansky, Handler and Medansky (1981) comment on the surprising paucity of psychodermatological literature. They divide dermatological patients into those whose complaint is part of a primary emotional disorder; those in whom an organic cutaneous problem influences the psychological state; and those in whom organic and emotional factors combine in different degrees to produce symptoms.

THE INFLUENCE OF THE EMOTIONAL STATE

A recent paper reports evidence that warts (skin reactions to a virus) may be induced by hypnosis (Gravitz, 1981). It has long been known that they can be cured by suggestion, if sufficiently prestigious. Atopic eczema, like its cousin childhood asthma, worsens not only with physical stimuli, but also in situations of emotional conflict; the liaison psychiatrist may be involved in alleviating the latter. A young married women developed patches of eczema on her fingers so that she had to remove her wedding ring whenever her critical mother-in-law came to stay. Contact dermatitis may also vary with the psychological state. A patient involved in a compensation suit against her employers, manufacturers of photographic materials, found that her hands — the subject of her claim — began to burn and weep on the day she as due to see either her solicitor or a doctor. Her skin could be seen to redden increasingly during an interview. Recurrences of herpes labialis and genitalis depend upon the activity of a resident virus, and a variety of factors, including emotional stress, may precipitate an attack (see Chapter 12). Psychological prophylaxis may be possible.

Blushing and patchy reddening on the neck and face, particularly on public and socially important occasions, are common in adolescence. If excessive and persistent they may be part of a social phobia, and respond best to phenelzine, relaxation therapy and exposure. Benzodiazepines and psychotherapy are of little use in this context. Rosacea tends to flare up under conditions of emotional tension, and so family or work-related conflicts need examination.

Psoriasis occurs often but not necessarily in patients with asthma, ulcerative colitis or rheumatoid arthritis — all diseases with psychomatic connotations. Exacerbations of psoriasis may coincide with anxiety-depressive symptoms but in manic-depressive patients the organic effect of lithium tends to make this skin condition worse. The prophylactic effects of lithium should not lightly be relinquished since a relapse into mania or depression may severely disrupt the patient's life.

SECONDARY EFFECTS OF SKIN DISORDERS

Disfiguring symptoms have emotional repercussions. Everyone knows the agony of an insecure adolescent with acne. If it persists, it may contribute towards social phobia, alcoholism or a paranoid state in the susceptible. Confidence-building cognitive and group therapy helps a distressed intractable sufferer.

Burns

Burns are traumatic physically and psychologically. Physiological shock and concern for survival are replaced by a series of psychological reactions culminating in a redefinition of identity and readjustment to life. In parallel, the patient's relatives are likely to be torn with sorrow, anger, guilt and frustration with his demandingness and the protracted time-scale for recovery (Goodstein, 1985). Multidisciplinary collaboration between social work, vocational rehabilitation, physiotherapy, medicine, surgery and psychiatry must begin long before discharge, and support must continue later. A psychiatrist may usefully hold the ring, and ensure that the family also receives the help it needs.

Dermatitis artefacta

Self-inflicted injuries range from the unthinking picking of the skin around the nails or of spots, in the insecure or tense person, to deliberate deep ulceration, its cause denied and concealed, for psychological reasons. Surgeons sometimes seek advice for patients whose wounds continually break down; they may be sterile or contaminated with faecal organisms. Cigarette burns and suction lesions can obviously only be self-inflicted where anatomically feasible, similarly with the application of irritant solutions. Munchausen-type psychopathy may be responsible, but schizophrenia or a depressive psychosis can also underlie self-mutilation. Other patients with masochistic, exhibitionist and aggressive tendencies may be neurotically depressed and seeking to attract love and care, or to escape from an intolerable life situation (Shafer and Shafer, 1980). Munchausen patients, manipulative, angry and pathetic, can be offered psychiatric outpatient follow-up; all other therapy is counterproductive. The other self-injuring patients require careful psychiatric assessment. Psychotics urgently need mediction; and neurotics an appraisal of their hopes, fears and emotional needs, so that they may be helped to cope with their current difficulties to find new goals and rewards. Confrontation, desired by non-psychiatric colleagues, has no place in the management of dermatitis artefacta. The correct diagnosis depends on the doctor's accepting the possibility of such behaviour despite denials, and accepting the patient as he is.

Dermatitis artefacta is not uncommon in cases of child abuse. Cigarette burns and other lesions occur, and the cause is denied. Jones (1983) describes a mother from a deprived and violent background who gouged lumps of skin from her baby's face and head. She showed the scars of similar lesions on her own arms and legs. The safety of the child is paramount in such cases, however convincing a parent may sound in his or her explanations.

Eczema

Children with eczema are deprived of the normal comfort of cuddling because it is painful, and their mothers feel distant and frustrated from their often screaming infant. Such parents need support.

Pruritis

This is a common symptom with many possible causes. Local causes include scabies, lice, insect bites, atopic and contact dermatitis, and urticaria. General causes are diabetes mellitus, thyroid disorders, nephritis, hepatic disease, gout, food allergy, leukaemia, Hodgkin's disease, carcinomatosis polycythaemia, rubra vera, age-related changes, and atrophic vaginitis. Anogenital itching may be due to haemorrhoids, discharge or sexual dissatisfaction (Musaph, 1976).

Delusions

Delusions associated with the skin are usually of dirt and infestation, and derive from tactile hallucinations. They occur in schizophrenia, paranoid depressive psychosis, organic brain states and cocaine psychosis (see Chapter 15). The calming and antipsychotic action of chlorpromazine is most useful in these cases, with tricyclic antidepressant also in depressives.

Scratching without itching

This is a self-grooming or masturbatory equivalent and manifests in situations of tension, such as trying to think of an answer, or having to wait at the traffic lights. Occasionally it develops into a compulsion with lichenification of the area affected.

INFECTIONS

Psychiatric symptoms in association with infections are sometimes prominent, causing diagnostic or management problems. Anxiety states are most likely in the prodrome and onset of the illness. Delirium may develop at the height of severe infection, and fatigue syndrome and sometimes frank depression may be sequelae.

Intracranial infections

These comprise encephalitis, meningitis (often both occur together) and brain abscess.

Acute encephalitis

Usually headache and irritability rapidly lead to prostration, confusion, perhaps delirium and fits, and finally coma. There are focal neurological signs including extensor plantar responses. The commonest type and that most likely to involve the psychiatrist is due to herpes simplex virus. This preferentially affects the temporal lobes and occasionally presents with bizarre behaviour, for instance sudden failure to recognise the spouse (Lishman, 1978). The delirious stage in this type of encephalitis may resemble delirium tremens, with vivid hallucinations and emotional overarousal. It is followed by intense retrograde amnesia, extending back over many months. Memory problems and parkinsonism may follow any encephalitis, but the most dramatic, encephalitis lethargica, is now encountered very rarely. However, a number of patients from the epidemics of 1918-20 and smaller outbreaks up to 1930 still remain in long-stay wards in psychiatric hospitals and are now part of psychogeriatric population. Acute encephalitis complicates mumps, measles and chicken pox, infectious hepatitis and mononucleosis, and in the United States and Russia there are still arthropod-borne epidemics of viral encephalitis.

Subacute encephalitis

Psychiatrists are more likely to be involved in the assessment and care of patients who may have mild benign encephalitic involvement. McEvedy and Beard (1973) saw and followed up a number of patients, predominantly adolescent girls, suffering from what was termed benign epidemic myalgic encephalomyelitis. The symptoms were of headache, fatigue, muscle pain and weakness, and lowered mood: perhaps viral in origin in some patients but hysterical in others (*British Medical Journal* Editorial, 1978). The symptoms of epidemic neuromyasthenia, described by Shelokov (1977), are similar: he believes them to be sequelae of infection with ECHO or Coxsackie viruses. Clinical depression requires treatment if present.

Slow viral infections.

Jakob-Creutzfeldt disease, spongiform encephalopathy, has been shown to be the result of an infection. A prodromal stage of several months is characterised by fatigue, insomnia, anxiety and depression; memory difficulties and weakness usher in accelerating intellectural deterioration, ataxia, progressive paralysis and death within two years. Amantidine 100 mg once or twice a day may be of some help in the early stages. The period between infection and the appearance of the disease is 15-20 years, so that those conducting post-mortem examinations on demented subjects must take particular precautions.

Meningitis

This characteristically produces severe headache, nuchal rigidity, photophobia and pyrexia. Lumbar puncture confirms the diagnosis. The only types of meningitis likely to involve the psychiatrist are syphilitic (Chapter 10) and tuberculous. The latter tends to come on insidiously in a child or adult with little or no neck stiffness or pyrexia and only transient headaches. Apathy, anorexia, sadness and an apparent change of personality are early manifestations, merging gently into memory impairment, clouded awareness and lack of activity. The pathognomonic symptoms and signs of meningitis supervene, and a stage of euphoria, confabulation and lasting amnesia may follow. It is in the early stages that the psychiatrist needs to be alert to the possibility of an infective process.

Cerebral abscess

This, too, may present deceptively and so involve psychiatric consultation. The patient may seem 'off colour' and headachey, mildly confused at times but often apyrexial and without focal neurological signs initially. Again, relatives may pick up a change of personality difficult to pinpoint. Frontal lobe abscess is particularly likely to present in this way; there may be unilateral anosmia. If chronic abscess if considered and there is no history of head injury, a source of infection should be sought, particularly in the lungs.

Other infective illness

Tropical infections such as trypanosomiasis, sandfly fever, dengue and malaria may all include cerebral involvement, and severe depression may be associated with them. Cysticercosis may also present with mental abnormalities. Typhoid causes delirium, and occasionally affective disorder as a sequel (Khosla *et al.* 1977).

Depression

This has long been considered to be a relatively frequent sequel to certain viral infections, in particular influenza, viral pneumonia infective hepatitis, and infectious mononucleosis (Cadie *et al.* 1976; Connolly, 1979). Sinanan and Hillary (1981), however, found little evidence for postinfluenzal clinical depression in a prospective study. Undoubtedly fatigue, both mental and physical, may linger on after such illnesses, and occasionally the patient feels suicidal, whatever the cause. The liaisonist must treat depression where he finds it. The illness may merely have been an added life event. Either a tricyclic or a more stimulating MAOI may be used. Imipramine 50-250 mg daily, or tranylcypromine 20-40 mg daily, are suitable.

Brucellosis and toxoplasmosis may be associated with severe depression as part of the illness rather than a sequel. They should be remembered when a young person suffers persistent unexplained symptoms of depression (Whitlock, 1982).

Bacterial pneumonia.

Often a disease of the elderly, chronically ill or alcoholic, bacterial pneumonia is particularly liable to produce delirium, partly because of poor cerebral oxygenation. Respiratory depression must be avoided as far as possible and the minimum sedation necessary for nursing management must be employed: small doses of haloperidol are suitable, for instance 1.5 mg twice a day and 3.5 mg at night (Schwab, 1980).

In vulnerable, usually old, patients, an acute organic brain syndrome can accompany almost any infection: urinary, gangrenous, pulmonary, or in the ear. A variable period of apparent dementia may follow the resolution of the acute mental state and infection. Time and patience are necessary, and in a substantial minority of cases mental recovery never becomes complete.

REFERENCES

British Medical Journal Editorial (1978) 'Epidemic Malaise', *British Medical Journal 1*, 1-2.

Cadie, M., Nye, F.J. and Storey, P. (1976) 'Anxiety and Depression after Infectious Mononucleosis', *British Journal of Psychiatry, 128*, 559-61

Connolly, J. (1979) 'Psychiatry in a General Hospital', in Hill, P., Murray, R. and Thorley, A. (Eds) *Essentials of Postgraduate Psychiatry*, Academic Press, London and New York

Goodstein, R.K. (1985) 'Burns: an Overview of Clinical Consequences Affecting Patients, Staff and Family', *Comprehensive Psychiatry, 26*, 43-57

Gravitz, M.A. (1981)'The Production of Warts by Suggestion as a Cultural Phenomenon', *American Journal of Clinical Hypnosis, 23*, 281-3

Jones, D.P.H. (1983) 'Dermatitis Artefacta in Mother and Baby as Child Abuse', *British Journal of Psychiatry, 143*, 199-200

Khosla, S.N., Srivastava, S.C. and Gupta, S (1977) 'Neuropsychiatric Manifestations of Typhoid', *Journal of Tropical Medicine and Hygiene, 80*, 85-98

Lishman, W.A. (1978) Chapter 8 in *Organic Psychiatry*, Blackwell, Oxford

McEvedy, C.P. and Beard, A.W. (1973) 'A Controlled Follow-up of Cases Involved in an Epidemic of Benign Myalgic Encephalomyelitis', *British Journal of Psychiatry, 122*, 141-50

Medansky, R.S., Handler, R.M. and Medansky, D.L. (1981) 'Self-evaluation of Acne and Emotion: a Pilot Study', *Psychosomatics*, 379-83

Musaph, H. (1976) 'Psychodermatology', in Hill, O.W. (Ed.) *Modern Trends in Psychosomatic Medicine — 3*, Butterworths, London

Schwab, J. (1980) 'Psychiatric Manifestations of Infectious Diseases', in Hall, R.C.W. (Ed.) *Psychiatric Presentations of Medical Illness*, Spectrum, New York

Shafer, N. and Shafer, R. (1980) 'Factitious Diseases Including Munchausen's Syndrome', *New York Journal of Medicine, 3*, 594-604

Shelokov, A. (1977) 'Epidemic Neuromyasthenia', in Hoeprich, P.D. (Ed.) *Infectious Diseases: a Modern Treatise of Infectious Processes*, Harper & Row, New York

Sinanan, K. and Hillary, I. (1981) 'Post-influenzal Depression', *British Journal of Psychiatry, 138*, 131-3

Whitlock, F.A. (1982) 'Infectious Diseases', in *Symptomatic Affective Disorders*, Academic Press, Sydney

13

Liaison in Oncology

Cancer — ' big C' — accounts for a quarter of deaths and is diagnosed in 700 000 Americans annually. At least one member is afflicted in two out of three families. No wonder that cancerphobia in which the patient is preoccupied with the thought that he has malignant disease, is common. Men are often obsessed by their bowel function, women with breast and gynaecological problems, doctors with query melanoma. The distressing idea of having cancer may arise as a symptom of endogenous depression, often associated with guilt, and sometimes achieving delusional strength. Suicide is a real risk. Treatment is urgent and is of the depression itself; it may include ECT or clomipramine infusions where these are available. In the US urgent, severe depression may be treated by intramuscular injections of amitriptyline 20-30 mg four times a day, changing to the oral route as soon as possible, usually after 24 hours. Neurotic and anxiety depressives may brood over the notion that they have cancer but are — at any rate temporarily — susceptible to and enjoy reassurance. The negative ideas of these patients recede also when the depression is treated. Particularly difficult to manage are the obsessional neurotics. These are the patients who go the rounds of hospitals and private clinics worrying over slight discrepancies in what they are told. If there is an element of depression, it is worth while to treat this, with clomipramine (30-100 mg daily), trazodone (50-200 mg daily) or an MAOI such as isocarboxazid (20-30 mg daily). Very occasionally a schizophrenic may hold the delusional belief that he has a cancer. This will respond as well as or as badly as his other psychotic symptoms to neuroleptic treatment. Physicians and sometimes surgeons invoke liaison psychiatry when faced with cancerphobic patients.

PSYCHIATRIC PRESENTATIONS OF MALIGNANT DISEASE

Whereas the cancerphobic feels desperate about what he does not have, other patients may complain initially of depression, conforming to either neurotic or psychotic patterns, but turn out to have cancer. In these patients fatigue is common: weariness and loss of enthusiasm for normally pleasurable activities without the sleep disturbance that characterises depression. Weight loss is likely. Whitlock (1978) in his study of suicides found that of 17 patients with cancer seven were not diagnosed until post-mortem, and so had not killed themselves in response to receiving the information. Depression may be analogous to carcinomatous neuropathy or myopathy; endocrine effects through a Cushing-like syndrome or hyperparathyroidism may induce depressive symptoms. Elderly men are especially prone to depression as the first manifestation of cancer. Pancreatic and colonic cancers have already been mentioned in this respect (see Chapter 7).

It has been suggested that not only may depression appear as the first warning of developing malignancy but it may be a facilitating, even causative, precursor. Galen (AD 131-200) hinted and Dr Guy (1759) said plainly that cancer was likelier in the melancholic; 100 years later James Paget in London and William Parker in America confirmed their view. A significant relationship between life stress and uterine cancer is demonstrated by Schmale and Iker (1966). Work in the last decade indicates that depression, and specifically bereavement, impairs immunocompetence, which is already waning at age 60 (Bartrop et al., 1977; Schleifer et al., 1983; Parkes, 1985). It is probable that neoplasia starts up frequently throughout life but is rapidly dispersed by the immune defences. An elderly depressive, particularly male, needs not only careful immediate screening for malignancy but also follow-up for several years even if this is negative — that is, if cancers are to be discovered early.

Case: Mrs L., 67, had been widowed and fell into a depression despite family support. Careful physical examination and investigation proved negative. Three months later her depression was responding to antidepressant therapy but she complained of difficulty with reading. By now she had mild papilloedema from cerebral secondaries from a primary bronchial carcinoma.

Brain tumour, either primary or metastatic, may present with any of a range of mental symptoms: irritability and depression are common, mania less so. Epileptic fits, listing to one side and headaches are frequent early symptoms.

The realistic suspicion of cancer from, for instance, finding a breast lump or noticing haematuria, induces immediate anxiety. Clinical anxiety and/or depression before biopsy is detectable in 40 per cent of breast cancer patients (Maguire, 1978). In fact only 8 per cent of them claim to have felt no anxiety on the discovery of a lump.

Cancer, once it is recognised, produces a multifaceted group of stressors:

1. emotional distress including depression, anger and anxiety: it is abnormal to have no reaction;
2. disruption to life activities and plans about work, family, social and sexual activity;
3. physical disability, direct and psychosomatic.

The long-established idea that schizophrenic patients are in some way protected from developing cancer is not borne out statistically (Masterson and O'Shea, 1984). Their reactions are often unemotional, however.

Telling patients their diagnosis in cancer cases calls for qualities in the physician and other staff that are conveyed clearly: concern, compassion, understanding and supportiveness. The patient must be told what he needs to know to accept treatment and rearrange his immediate future, within what he can tolerate at the time. He may well reject information that he has requested by showing signs of irritability, cutting short the conversation, or — frequently — erasing from his mind the unwelcome news. Several discussions are needed, during which the patient will indicate his readiness or otherwise to receive a definite diagnosis of cancer: he may never wish to know for certain. On the other hand patients are sensitive and skilful at picking up medical anxiety from non-verbal signals and unconscious innuendo, as so chillingly portrayed by Solzhenitsyn in *Cancer Ward*.

PSYCHOLOGICAL IMPACT OF A DIAGNOSIS OF CANCER

Maguire (1985) delineates the specific areas of concern of the cancer patient as uncertainty, with anxiety exacerbating and subsiding with each follow-up appointment; helplessness in modifying the course of the disease by personal effort, unlike, for instance adhering to a diet in hypertension, diabetes and heart disease; a usually fruitless search for meaning — whom or what to blame; a sense of stigma and personal failure; and isolation since friends and relatives are embarrassed and uncertain about whether it is kind or cruel to ask the patient about the progress of his disease (Rassidakis *et al.*, 1978; Whitlock, 1982).

These are logical conclusions. However, Cassileth *et al.* (1984) in an authoritative study of 758 patients with chronic disease, in six diagnostic groups, found that those with diabetes, dermatological disorders, arthritis, renal disease or cancer did not differ significantly from each other or from the population at large in mental health, but all scored considerably better than a group of depressives under treatment. In all groups patients with recently diagnosed illness scored worse on the Mental Health Index (MHI) than those diagnosed for four months or more. The MHI addresses feelings and behaviours in the previous month and comprises five subscales including anxiety and depression. Higher age was associated with better MHI scores, independent of diagnosis, indicating better adaptation to illness. The natural tendency is not borne out to infer a direct relation between psychological status and such factors as loss of mobility, dependence on drugs or medical technology and physical discomfort. Subjective perceptions of personal circumstances and handicap are of prime importance. Somewhat similar conclusions are reached by Funch and Marshall (1983) in their 20-year study of the role of stress, social support and age in survival of breast cancer cases.

Quality of life is currently and fashionably a matter of concern to surgeons and physicians dealing with cancer (Clark and Fallowfield, 1986). Characteristically they prefer such rigid measures as rating scales for assessing their patients' distress, sprinkled with highly subjective 'common sense' involving such items as work, weakness and sexual competence. Our sympathies are aroused, but in fact patients like other human beings have remarkable mechanisms for adjustment: witness the response of the citizens of Beirut to daily danger and privation. For effective adaptation to adversity, the most important factor is the patient's sense of self-worth, something integral to his personality and often associated with the feeling of being loved or appreciated for himself; this does not feature in questionnaires.

Most patients adjust within a few months to a major change in their health and reasonable future expectations. Their relatives, friends and colleagues adapt also. Medical and nursing help is accepted at best on a partnership basis, involving trust. Apart from ongoing specialist nursing advice in ileostomy, colostomy or haemodialysis cases, it is usually better not to intervene by offering counselling and emotional support. To neuroticise the patient and encourage his dependency on a professional may delay and deflect him from developing a workable co-operative effort with those of lasting significance in his life. In our study of breast cancer patients we found only two in 54 who were clinically anxious or depressed and requiring treatment, and both had major personal problems (Bulman and Gomez, 1986). Although the psychiatrist must be ready to offer help to any oncology patient who needs it because of functional or organic psychopathology, it is often the staff of a cancer ward who really need support.

Mental attitude

What appears to be of paramount importance in the prognosis of breast cancer at least is the patient's coping style. This may include denial of the seriousness of her situation, a fighting spirit, stoic acceptance of disease, or a helpless-hopeless stance. Either of the latter two responses is associated with shortened survival. The only additional factor making a significant difference to survival is histological tumour type; age, menopausal status, clinical stage, tumour size, surgery and radiotherapy appear to have little influence on outcome (Pettingale, 1984). It is the liaison psychiatrist who will be expected to attempt to alter or improve mental attitudes. Unlike the situation in an incontrovertibly terminal case, there must be no attempt, if there is any hope of remission, to break down a defence of denial (Meyerowitz et al., 1983).

Selective denial which allows compliance with treatment is an adaptation which serves some patients well for years following diagnosis and treatment. Other patients prefer to confront the situation, redefine their life problems, and use a flexible range of coping mechanisms. They are likely to indicate when and where they require particular support. Although submission to disease is not to be recommended, some patients find strength in meditation. Magarey (1983), an Australian professor of surgery, advocates this approach as an adjunct to physical and social measures. In his view ' . . . to be most effective it is the therapist who should meditate' and then transfer his calm and contentment to the patient. Not all patients or therapists could embrace this or any other faith, but it might be of particular benefit to the parents of children with terminal cancer, either at home or in hospital (Kohler and Radford, 1985).

The multifunded research into malignancy has resulted in enhanced life expectancy for patients — at the cost of enduring physical treatment that may be unpleasant and frightening and have aversive side-effects. One role of liaison psychiatry is to help patients to put up with therapy that may be life-saving (Burish and Lyles, 1983).

SURGERY

This is the first line of attack in many cancers, for instance uterine, breast, colorectal and laryngeal. Major problems arise when the effects of treatment challenge normal social and sexual functioning. When breast cancer is treated by mastectomy it is well known to impair self-image and induce the fear, often justified, that the mutilation will be offputting to men. Sexuality is also disturbed (Gerard, 1983). Some women delay telling their doctors about a breast lump for fear of mastectomy, and internal prostheses often cause anxiety. Maguire found that counselling *per se* before and after surgery was of no help to breast cancer patients, except that those needing psychiatric help were referred on and benefited in 88 per cent of cases (Maguire, 1978; Maguire *et al*, 1980). By far the best ploy is for surgeons to restrict themselves to lumpectomy, with follow-on radiotherapy. Psychiatric morbidity among lumpectomy patients at the Westminster Hospital in London is slight, temporary and usually associated with unrelated life events if it reaches clinical intensity. Steinberg *et al.* (1985) report a better sexual and overall adaptation to lumpectomy than to mastectomy in a comparative trial.

A secondary effect of breast surgery involving axillary clearance is lymphoedema and reduced mobility of the arm on the affected side.

> *Case*: Mrs C.H., 47, had an unhappy marriage and enjoyed her work as a waitress. After mastectomy she developed lymphoedema in her left arm and could no longer carry trays. There has been no recurrence of disease over the last 13 years but Mrs C.H. has had several convictions for shoplifting since her operation. She blames her 'bad arm'.

Impaired sexual functioning may be a direct result of adrenalectomy, and bladder or prostate surgery, but more commonly arises after pelvic surgery because of psychological trauma. Gynaecological surgery ranges from hysterectomy to radical vulvectomy; apart from direct surgical effects such as shortening of the vagina, the patient's libido and capacity for orgasm may be markedly reduced. Partners are sometimes superstitiously afraid of contracting cancer by contact. Anything involving the genital area can be intensely upsetting.

Case : R.G., 41, had undergone successful unilateral orchidec-
tomy for malignancy while a naval officer. Fifteen years later, having left the services, he longed to settle and marry, but felt he was
'only half a man'. When an affectionate girlfriend uncovered the
situation, he was humiliated and hanged himself.

The main problems are psychosexual with urinary and colorectal
cancer surgery involving ostomy (see Chapter 7).

Surgery for head and neck malignancy can have devastating effects
on appearance, swallowing and speaking. Special help with communication skills and repair for the self-esteem are urgently needed.
The Lost Cord Society helps laryngectomees in the United States.

CHEMOTHERAPY

In contrast to the situation in the 1960s when this was a last resort,
it is now a commonplace ongoing treatment for cancer, promising
cure for some. Indeed tamoxifen has recently been suggested as a
prophylactic against breast cancer in those at particular risk. The effect
of cytotoxic drugs, the usual chemotherapeutic agents, on normal
tissues produces such side-effects as vomiting, diarrhoea, hair loss
(particularly distressing to women), change in skin colour, temporary
or persisting impotence or frigidity, and such negative emotions as
depression and anxiety. All of these, including the last two, are direct
pharmacological results. In addition some patients develop conditioned
responses such as anxiety, nausea and vomiting to reminders of the
therapy, even mental. Antiemetics are of limited value and may have
side-effects of their own; behavioural interventions including hypnosis, autohypnosis, systematic desensitisation and biofeedback help
some patients. Counselling is of no use (Morrow and Morrell, 1982),
and some patients condition to relaxation procedures, exacerbating
the problem since they feel nauseous as they think of the key phrases.

REVERSE BARRIER NURSING

Reverse barrier nursing by which the patient is confined to a germ-
free atmosphere, isolated from skin-to-skin contact, may be required
when chemotherapy reduces immunity drastically, as in some forms
of leukaemia. With support from staff, family and friends, patients
in protective isolation — including children — do not appear to suffer

any increase in psychological distress (Kellerman *et al.*, 1980).

RADIOTHERAPY

Fifty per cent of cancer patients receive some form of radiation therapy, but, like chemotherapy, it may have severe side-effects. Indeed, the combination of chemotherapy and radiotherapy is thought, rarely, to induce acute leukaemia as a late event especially in Hodgkin's disease, breast and ovarian cancers and multiple myeloma (Whitehouse, 1985). The usual, more immediate troubles vary with the area irradiated and include fatigue, skin irritation, burns, and local hair loss. Nausea and vomiting arise with treatment of the abdomen or any large area. Abdominal and pelvic irradiation may cause diarrhoea, sexual dysfunction and sterility. Adequate explanation and preparation are particularly necessary with radiotherapy: the apparatus itself is intimidating. Relaxation training and other methods used to avoid or combat side-effects from chemotherapy may be of some use in radiotherapy, and there is evidence that psychotherapy during radiotherapy benefits not only emotional status but physical symptoms namely fatigue, anorexia, nausea and vomiting (Forester *et al.*, 1985). Men in particular benefit, presumably because they are normally less able to ventilate their emotions.

TERMINATION OF TREATMENT

Termination of a course of treatment, however unpleasant that treatment might be, may bring its own problems. Patients often miss the camaraderie and the routine of coming for treatment. Various voluntary associations offer help but companionship is difficult to arrange.

PSYCHIATRIC MORBIDITY

Anxiety, depression, even despair may engulf young adult cancer patients in particular. To them it seems grossly unfair that they are stricken. Because their will and wish for life had been naturally high, with illness and death seen as remote, fear and anger are more acute in these patients. Children, dependent as they are on adults to look after them, are less severely distressed, and the elderly can more easily accommodate to ill-health. Patients who are depressed and also physically and emotionally frail while undergoing treatment may respond to antidepressants. It is important to make two checks before starting them: first to make sure that hepatic function is adequate to metabolise psychotropic medication; secondly by tactful mental assessment to exclude cerebral organicity. With cerebral metastases or electrolyte abnormalities, antidepressants are likely to precipitate an acute organic brain syndrome. Apart from these circumstances it is helpful to prescribe a stimulating antidepressant if the patient complains of deadly fatigue: an MAOI is ideal unless it is contraindicated because of narcotic analgesia, in which case imipramine (30-100 mg daily, divided) or clomipramine (30-150 mg daily divided, where available) may be used. In those who are agitated, amitriptyline (30-150 mg/24 hours), doxepin (30-100 mg/24 hours) or trazodone (50-250 mg/24 hours) may be given. Psychotherapy is useful but labour intensive, and simple counselling is worthwhile mainly for practical problems. Hypnotherapy and relaxation techniques help patients to cope with pain, tension and difficulties in sleeping.

Some patients puzzle the oncologists by the severity of their pain, weakness or incapacity for self-care. Careful assessment may reveal that they are afraid to leave the shelter of hospital, or they fear their spouses will leave them alone and afraid, or they are angry with relatives and others who do not have cancer, or there are particular activities or 'duties' they wish to avoid. These patients need time, affection and support, then encouragement. Confrontation is counterproductive and drugs do not help.

ORGANIC BRAIN SYNDROMES

Organic brain syndromes are obviously likely in cancer patients from disturbances in calcium, urea and electrolyte levels, hepatic dysfunction and cerebral metastases. The most useful drugs are haloperidol, chlorpromazine and chlormethiazole, and, in emergency disturbance, droperidol, which has a short action (see Chapter 3).

REFERENCES

Bartrop, R.W., Lazarus, L., Luckhurst, E., Kiloh, L.G. and Penny, R. (1977) 'Depressed Lymphocyte Function after Bereavement', *Lancet, 1*, 834-6
Bulman, A. and Gomez, J. (1986) 'Psychological Response to Lumpectomy and Radiotherapy in the First Year,' awaiting publication.

Burish, T.G. and Lyles, J.M. (1983) 'Coping with the Adverse Effects of Cancer Treatments', in Burish T.C. and Bradley, L.A. (Eds) *Coping with Chronic Disease*, Academic Press, New York

Cassileth, B.R., Lusk, E.K., Strouse, T.B., Miller, D.S., Brown, L.L., Cross, P.A. and Tenaglia, A.N. (1984) 'Psychosocial Status in Chronic Illness', *New England Journal of Medicine, 311*, 506-11

Clark, A. and Fallowfield, L.J. (1986) 'Quality of Life Measurements in Patients with Malignant Disease: a Review', *Journal of the Royal Society of Medicine, 79*, 165-9

Forester, B., Kornfeld, D.S. and Fleiss, J.L. (1985) 'Psychotherapy during Radiotherapy: Effects on Emotional and Physical Distress', *American Journal of Psychiatry, 142*, 22-7

Funch, D.P. and Marshall, J. (1983) 'The Role of Stress, Social Support and Age in Survival from Breast Cancer', *Journal of Psychosomatic Research, 27*, 77-83

Gerard, D.M. (1983) 'Thirty years Review: Mastectomy and Sexual Functioning', *British Journal of Sexual Medicine, 109*, 22-28

Guy, R. (1759) *An Essay on Schirrous Tumors and Cancer*, Churchill, London

Kellerman, J., Siegel, S. and Rigler, D. (1980) 'Special Treatment Modalities: Laminar Airflow Rooms', in Kellerman, J. (Ed.) *Psychological Aspects of Childhood Cancer*, C.C. Thomas, Springfield, Illinois

Kohler, J.A. and Radford, M. (1985) 'Terminal Care for Children Dying of Cancer: Quantity and Quality of life', *British Medical Journal, 291*, 115-16

Magarey, C. (1983) 'Holistic Cancer Therapy', *Journal of Psychosomatic Research, 27, ,* 181-4

Maguire, P. (1978) 'The Psychological and Social Sequelae of Mastectomy', in Howells, J.G. (Ed.) *Modern Perspectives in the Psychiatric Aspects of Surgery*, Macmillan, London

Maguire, P. (1985) 'The Psychological Impact of Cancer', *British Journal of Hospital Medicine, 34*, 100-3

Maguire, P., Tait, A., Brook, M., Thomas, C. and Sellwood, R. (1980) 'Effect of Counselling on the Psychiatric Morbidity Associated with Mastectomy', *British Medical Journal, 281*, 1454-6

Masterson, E. and O'Shea, B. (1984) 'Smoking and Malignancy in Schizophrenia', *British Journal of Psychiatry, 145*, 429-32

Meyerowitz, B.E., Heinrich, R.L. and Schah, C.C. (1983) 'A Competency-based Approach to Coping with Cancer', in Burish, T.G. and Bradley, L.A. (Eds) *Coping with Chronic Disease*, Academic Press, New York

Morrow, G.R. and Morrell, C. (1982) 'Behavioural Treatment for the Anticipatory Nausea and Vomiting Induced by Cancer Chemotherapy', *New England Journal of Medicine, 307*, 1476-80

Parkes, C.M. (1985) 'Bereavement', *British Journal of Psychiatry, 146*, 11-17

Pettingale, K.W. (1984) 'Coping and Cancer Prognosis', *Journal of Psychosomatic Research, 28*, 363-4

Rassidakis, N.C, Erocritou, A. and Volidou, M. (1978) 'The Psychopathology of Cancer', in Howells, J.G. (Ed.) *Modern Perspectives in the Psychiatric Aspects of Surgery*, Macmillan, London

Schleifer, S.J., Keller, S.E., Camerino, M., Thornton, J.C. and Stein, M. (1983) 'Suppression of Lymphocyte Stimulation Following Bereavement',

Journal of the American Medical Association, 250, 374-7

Schmale, A.H. and Iker, H.P. (1966) 'The Psychological Setting of Uterine Cancer', *Annals of New York Academy of Science, 125*, 807-13

Steinberg, M.D., Juliano, M.A. and Wise, L. (1985) 'Psychological Outcome of Lumpectomy versus Mastectomy in the Treatment of Breast Cancer', *American Journal of Psychiatry, 142*, 34-9

Whitehouse, J.M.A. (1985) 'Risk of Leukaemia Associated with Cancer Chemotherapy', *British Medical Journal, 290*, 261-3

Whitlock, F.A. (1978) 'Suicide, Cancer and Depression', *British Journal of Psychiatry, 132*, 269-74

Whitlock, F.A. (1982) 'Cancer and Depression', in *Symptomatic Affective Disorders*, Academic Press, Sydney

14

Terminal Illness

Death is inevitable and is increasingly likely to occur in a hospital, hospice or nursing home. Even in the 1960s and 1970s, only 20 per cent of people died at home, and the trend is for this number to diminish (Flynn and Stewart, 1979). For the sick patient, death is the least desirable outcome and for the professionals it feels like failure. The relatives are caught up in and react to the final drama, however muted and modified. The psychiatrist can help all three — patient, professionals, relatives — through the process and its aftermath. Because of medical technology the trajectory of dying is often a longer, flatter curve. This lengthens the period of strain and apparently fruitless labour, but also allows time for adjustment by everyone concerned and the most beneficial management. Indeed the most difficult and unsatisfactory ways of dying are those that happen in haste, in the harshly clinical setting of an intensive therapy unit.

MEDICAL AND PHYSIOLOGICAL ASPECTS OF DYING

Pain

Pain, agonising, intractable and intensifying, is the major fear in most people's perception of dying. It may be insignificant in pulmonary disease, and easily managed in cardiovascular and gastroenterological disorders (Petrich and Holmes, 1980). Even in malignant disease, pain is not always present, but when it is it is exhausting and demoralising and must be adequately controlled.

An accurate diagnosis of the cause of pain is essential, and a review of the subject has been made in Chapter 3. An important factor in terminal illness is that the dangers of addiction do not apply, and whatever dosage of analgesia is necessary to alleviate pain should be given. Excessive amounts may make the patient unpleasantly dopey or nauseous, however. Pain causes particular anxiety for a cancer patient, who may for instance, misinterpret pain of muscular spasm for metastasis. Complaints of pain may be maintained because of the patient's fear of being discharged home, where help is amateur; or his distress and anger at his plight may be displaced on to the doctor, whom he can blame for mismanaging his continuing pain.

In most cases, however, pain can be held within tolerable limits by medication: analgesics, neuroleptics and perhaps an antidepressant that increases available serotonin such as clomipramine (30-150 mg daily) or trazodone (50-200 mg daily). Clomipramine may not be available in the US and perhaps a tricyclic antidepressant such as imipramine may be used. Haloperidol in doses of 1.5-5 mg is the best neuroleptic if the patient prefers to feel clear-headed; chlorpromazine in 25-75 mg doses if he welcomes sedation. Morphine and its derivatives act at many neural levels affecting the sensory, emotional and cognitive aspects of pain and reducing arousal (Levy, 1983).

Weakness

Weakness is common in the dying and calls for the 'TL' of 'tender loving care' to sugar the pill of involuntary dependency. It is a privilege for the carer to be allowed to help, whether spouse or nurse, and the rags of dignity must be respected.

Dyspnoea and cough

These are made worse by and in turn enhance anxiety. Benzodiazepine anxiolytics, especially diazepam, theoretically depress respiration, but in practice improve breathing in the very anxious. Relaxation therapy and breathing exercises may be helpful, and in continued distress opiate, cocaine and neuroleptic draughts, such as the Brompton mixture, provide physical and psychological ease.

Anorexia

Both patients and relatives are often afraid that missing a meal means immediate disaster. Both need reassurance, and the patient should be encouraged to eat a little or a lot, as he wishes. This is one area where he can still exercise choice and control. Fluid intake must, of course, be maintained.

Nausea and vomiting

These may be a reaction to medication, symptomatic of disease or a manifestation of anxiety — hence the expression 'sick with fear'. Haloperidol starting at 1.5 mg t.d.s. before meals, is anxiolytic and antinauseant; phenothiazines such as prochlorperazine (5 mg, three times daily) or chlorpromazine (25-50 mg, three times daily) may be used if sedation is desired. Autohypnosis helps with vomiting partly emotionally associated with treatment.

Paralysis

The indignity of needing help to move or wash is devastating if it has come on suddenly. Unless the patient has happily regressed, he or she should be treated with professional competence rather than familiarity. All that can be said to increase his confidence and self-esteem should be voiced. Paralysed patients are often angry with the part that will not move and should be enabled to express and discuss such feelings.

An explanation for physical symptoms should be simple and factual, avoiding alarm-signal phrases. A 'type of cancer' strikes less of a chill than baldly saying 'cancer', and 'a small area of affected tissue' — however unfortunately situated — is not so recognisably deadly as 'secondary spread'. Euphemisms are not used to deceive but to allow the patient time to prepare for unwelcome information.

PSYCHOLOGICAL ASPECTS OF TERMINAL ILLNESS

Kubler-Ross (1970) divides the natural history of dying into five stages, starting with the patient's initial realisation of his situation, spoken or otherwise:

(1)   denial and isolation
(2)   anger
(3)   bargaining
(4)   depression
(5)   acceptance

Clearly this progression takes time.

Dame Cicely Saunders, pioneer of the hospice movement, writes reassuringly '... death is almost always preceded by a perfect willingness to die' (Saunders, 1966). It is likely that those applying and accepted for admission to a hospice are already wishing to learn such a state of mind. Others confront death with fear or defiance to the end. Nor does every patient go through all five phases delineated by Kubler-Ross. The very old who have lived out a long life can more easily relinquish what is left: it is interesting that they are more likely to do so just after their birthdays or Christmas Day. Those weary with protracted and tedious illness, especially if there is pain, may welcome death, as may the severely depressed or those with an unresolved bereavement reaction who may prefer not to go on alone. It is adults of under 50, previously fit, whose lives are full of present activity and the promise of much to come, who feel it is unfair and intolerable to have everything taken from them.

Denial

In what Pattison (1977) calls the crisis of knowledge of death to come, denial is a mechanism for avoiding overwhelming anxiety, and for continuing for the time being with near normal living. The patient may keep his thoughts to himself for fear that someone may challenge them, frail as they are; he is isolated both by doubts he dare not express and denial that may not be believed. He may force himself into phrenetic activity to demonstrate that he is all right, or he may, in the face of the evidence, go out of his way to explain to others the trivial nature of his problems. Denial fulfils a useful function — temporarily. It should not be broken down until the patient gives some indication that he is ready to relinquish it, or unless anxiety is clearly showing through.

Some patients ask earnestly to be told the truth; but this may not mean that they are prepared emotionally to hear the worst. A sign of unreadiness is asking a junior nurse or medical student for information; this can be discounted as without authority if it is not what was hoped for. Other patients show sudden irritability or unease if, after all, they cannot yet face inescapable facts. To compel a patient to consider his prognosis too soon is cruel and incidentally removes any faintest hope that his clinical course will take an upturn. At all stages the honest reassurance can be given that whatever happens the patient will not have to struggle alone: professionals exist for the sole purpose of providing help when it is needed.

Denial can be counterproductive when it has become threadbare, and then the greater relief obtains from talking openly about prognosis and associated practical problems. Relatives are sometimes loath for the patient to know his situation: this may be a vicarious form of denial and they may need supportive persuasion to lower their guard and share more fully the patient's experience.

Anger

Anger usually follows denial in the reaction to approaching death. Few are ready to die and the normal mechanism for coping with danger — in war, from muggers, or infectious disease — is to assume that other people, only, will be victims. When the worst is realised, a common complaint is 'Why me? What have I done to deserve this?' Even a heavy smoker, struck with bronchial disease, will point to others who smoked much more and got away with it. Whereas anyone can sympathise with a patient's anger at being ill, it sometimes goes unrecognised when it is displaced. Doctors, nurses and other staff often come in for displaced anger — nothing about the patient's care is right! Bitter complaints about noise are not uncommon from patients who sleep 20 hours of the 24. Relatives also may come into the fire of criticism, particularly when a patient is at home for weekends.

It is worth explaining to any who may be hurt by a patient's expressions of anger where the blame really belongs. Similarly, relatives in their distress may turn on each other: child against father, mother against daughter-in-law, etc.

Bargaining

Those accustomed to pray, those who do so only in extreme circumstance and those who profess no faith at all, or atheism, are all likely to go through this stage. It is an unwilling step towards the inevitability of giving up everything. 'If I could live long enough to see my first grandchild, to have Christmas at home, to see Venice . . . ' Often a foolhardy trip is arranged and it may be achieved at some cost to whoever is helping the patient.

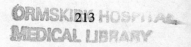

Depression

Sadness is universal when so many losses are in prospect: loss of occupation and status, of dearest relatives and friends, of ambitions and belongings, of strength and independence, and perhaps of the ability to think clearly. Bodily malfunctions and sometimes smell, loss of hair and deteriorated appearance add to a patient's humiliation. Continued pain is lowering. Clinical depression requires treatment and is considered later, but the normal sadness of parting with life calls for understanding companionship and for permission to talk about fears, regrets and others feelings as often as it is a relief. The opinions and practical suggestions of a dying person should be treated as seriously as if he were well: he needs to feel that he is a valued member of the living world as long as he is available (Hinton, 1980).

Acceptance

This goal may be reached by various routes, and is easier to achieve if the patient has had some experience of other people's death, even that of another occupant of the ward. It is reassuring to see such a person cared for and supported, including the use of medication (Steadford, 1984).

PSYCHIATRIC COMPLICATIONS

A range of emotional reactions is normal in terminal illness, and organic effects, subtle or severe, iatrogenic or due to disease, may also produce psychological changes. The patient's mental state may become, in itself, a cause for concern and fall within the parameters of a clinical psychiatric disorder requiring attention.

Anxiety

Anxiety is inevitable. Death is a once-only experience, new for everyone and with no-one to say subjectively that it was easy. Anxiety awakens at the first hint of something sufficiently wrong to consult the doctor. It advances when simple — or dramatic and surgical — treatment fails to restore health. Most patients in their private moments allow their imagination to extrapolate to disastrous dyscontrol and an agonising end. Panic may break through protective denial early on, or increase insidiously. Separation anxiety, fear of suddenly dying alone, and fear of rejection all respond to the reassurance of close company and communication.

Anxiety in the clinical range may cause insomnia, nightmares, restlessness, nausea and vomiting, frequent motions and micturition, breathlessness and sharpening of pain. Relaxation therapy with physical and psychological strands should be given in person initially, and the patient given an audiotape to follow on. It is, of course, easier just to give sedating drugs such as lorazepam (1-2.5 mg doses), diazepam (2-5 mg doses), haloperidol (0.5-5 mg doses) or chlorpromazine (25-50 mg doses). Diazepam is an excellent muscle relaxant but a respiratory depressant with prolonged action; it is useful in acute anxiety.

Depression

Depression as a clinical disorder involves self-blame, hopelessness, lack of responsiveness and often a lack of co-operation with treatment and suicidal ideas. Suppression of anger may produce depression in Kubler-Ross's stage 2. In terminal care the patient's state of health distorts the phenomenology of depression. If the patient has no difficulty in sleeping, this may be a measure of his exhaustion, despite depression. On the other hand, anorexia and anergy may be symptomatic of physical but not psychological disease. It is pathognomonic of depression if the patient does not want to see his visitors.

The reasons for clinical depression may be situational, the effect of pain or of non-metastatic effects of malignancy, or iatrogenic from sedating drugs, corticosteroids, analgesics, cytotoxics or radiotherapy. To enable the easy communication necessary for psychotherapy, antidepressant medication may be necessary. If opiates are not required the most rapid and effective lift of mood is achieved with tranylcypromine (10-40 mg) or phenelzine (15-60 mg) in the early part of the day and trimipramine (10-75 mg) at night. When narcotic analgesics are being given, non-MAOI antidepressants are used. Clomipramine is the best when pain is a problem. It is stimulating in low dosage and calming and more effectively antidepressant in high dosage. It is usually given by mouth, but starter doses of 25 mg intramuscularly twice a day may be helpful in grossly unresponsive patients, or a course of intravenous infusions in the severely depressed. Where clomipramine is not available, as may be the case in the US, imipramine or amitriptyline may be given, in daily dosage of 50-150 mg. One or two intramuscular doses of 20 mg may be used with either of these drugs if a rapid response is urgent — because of suicidally severe depression or refusal to take nourishment. Amitriptyline is the standard effective antidepressant, immediately sedating but taking seven days to reach a mood-elevating result however it is given. Meanwhile constipation and dry mouth may be troublesome. Maprotiline, a tetracyclic, is appropriate for neurotic depressives; trazodone or doxepin for the anxious: maprotiline and doxepin are given in daily — or nightly — doses of 50-200 mg; trazodone 50-250 mg. Those whose depression has a paranoid flavour should also receive trifluoperazine 1 mg b.d. or take thioridazine as their antidepressant. This drug is also preferred if the patient is confused: tricyclics make matters worse. Thioridazine should be given in daily/nightly dosage of 50-125 mg.

Suicide

Suicidal ideas are common, and suicide is an appreciable risk in terminal disease. Four per cent of suicides in Bristol were found to have disease likely to have been fatal within six months, and Hinton (1972) found that 16 per cent of referrals to him of terminal disorders arose after a suicide attempt. Some patients are suffering a clinical depression; others find realistically that life is no longer worthwhile; a few are altruistic (Selby, 1985). In acutely suicidal depression, electroconvulsive therapy is not contraindicated because of terminal status and may alter the patient's affect miraculously. More often a mixture of sedation and antidepressant medication and undemanding warmth achieves the same result in a week or two.

Personality change

The chief complainant of this is likely to be a relative. An outgoing or thoughtful or good-humoured man or woman may become introvert, selfish, suspicious and irritable or continually complaining. The formerly independent person may become even more dependent than is physically appropriate, and peevish with it. Such changes in the face of lethal disease are understandable and usually represent a depressive illness, calling for treatment. The relatives need support also, and not all of them have had a rewarding relationship with the patient even in the past.

Conversion hysteria

A patient who is dying may still express his anxieties in conversion symptoms: mutism or hysterical coma. Time, reassurance and a small regular dose of diazepam (2-5 mg doses) or hypnosis will restore the *status quo*.

Hypomania

Euphoria may be induced by steroids or other organic upset, and occasionally a manic rather than a depressive reaction will arise. In either case haloperidol is the drug of choice for symptomatic control of excitement while the possible causes are investigated. Oral or parenteral dosage will be 5-20 mg three or four times daily, usually.

Paranoid states

Paranoid states in which the patient believes the medication is making him worse, that there are plots on the ward, or that the doctors are arranging his murder are often organic, but may be due to severe anxiety or a functional psychosis. Again haloperidol is the safest first choice of medication. In these cases smaller doses, for instance 1.5 mg two or three times daily, are sometimes adequate.

Organic brain syndromes

Acute and subacute confusional states commonly come and go in terminal disease, especially in the elderly. Naturally primary or secondary cerebral tumours or cerebrovascular accidents may produce gross organic symptomatology. Usually the cause is obvious, but electroencephalography or CT scan may be called for. Fluctuant consciousness and disorientation, particularly in regard to time, motor restlessness and rambling talk, persecutory delusions or complete withdrawal are typical manifestations of organicity, and are usually worse at night. If there is no indication of structural disruption, physiological abnormalities should be sought: dehydration, hypoxia, hypoglycaemia, unusual levels of electrolytes, calcium or magnesium. Medication should be reviewed in the search for treatable causes. Neuroleptic medication increasing in the evening and at night, and constant reassurance and reorientation are required (Davidson, 1981).

Fifty seven per cent of dying patients become confused during their illness, whereas the remaining 43 per cent are able to concentrate and think clearly until the last 24-48 hours. Some patients welcome the drowsy, dreamy state induced by analgesia and sedation, and others dislike feeling muddled. It is important to tailor the medication to the patient's preference.

Children

A child's impending death is particularly upsetting to relatives and to professional staff. Young children live intensely in the present, and although they can appreciate the meaning of death from about age three, disappointment about all they will miss has less impact. Similarly, they have less of the past to regret, and the regression and dependency brought about by their illness comes more naturally to children than adults. Children learn fear from older people, and equally have confidence in the adults' power to protect them, so long as they present as confident and competent as well as caring. Children are essentially realists and in a long terminal illness their personal priorities readjust so that the hierarchy of important people may run: nurses, doctors, ancillary staff, parents, siblings and friends. Parents may be hurt by their child's lack of welcome when they visit and the situation needs explaining. It also provides a chance for the parents to give much-needed care to their other children and to each other. A sick child throws an enormous strain on family relationships; the guilt and anger generated by the situation may be projected on to the other partner or grandparents or vice versa. Psychotherapy with the family is the most valuable task the liaison psychiatrist can undertake or directly delegate.

THE PSYCHIATRIST'S ROLE IN TERMINAL ILLNESS

The role of the psychiatrist in terminal illness is:

(a) to help the multidisciplinary therapeutic team to observe and respond to the patient's psychological needs in the various stages of his illness, and to deal with complications as they arise;

(b) to help the relatives understand and react appropriately to the patient's changing state;

(c) to support the multidisciplinary team and help them to cope with their own feelings of failure and of sadness, and to facilitate the expression of views about management as well as feelings in staff meetings;

(d) to support directly or indirectly, the relatives during the patient's illness and when he dies.

General principles of the care of the dying

Pain must quickly be brought under control. Clinical anxiety and depression and organic brain syndromes require drug therapy as well as psychotherapeutic alleviation.

Psychotherapy is probably beneficial to most patients in their final illness, and for some is essential to ameliorate distress. The aims are to restore and preserve the patient's dignity and self-worth and a measure of control over his life. A course must be steered between confrontation and being patronising. Sobel (1981) advocates what he calls cognitive-behavioural thanatology, emphasising the choices still available to the patient, whereas Redd (1982) prefers a more strictly behavioural approach. Pleasant and positive statements by the patient are rewarded by the company of relatives or nurses, whereas excessive complaints lead to a reduction in time spent with him. This ploy is said to reduce the patient's awareness of pain since it is no longer the main method by which he can attract care and sympathy. By contrast, the psychotherapy of Shneidman (1978) involves breaking the traditional patient/therapist barrier and entering into a real relationship with the patient, albeit time-limited. This approach gives the patient a new, positive experience of friendship to set against the negative factors.

Joint psychotherapy with the key relative or partner and the patient can allow honest exchanges in the safe situation of having a mediator: misunderstandings, fears and feelings of guilt can be worked out. This is also a time to try to avoid or put right, by better understanding, jealousies and mistrust between different family factions. It is not unusual for a young adult, in terminal illness, to turn to his mother rather than his wife or partner: the latter needs support and explanation.

HOSPICE CARE

There is a growing movement towards nursing the terminally ill in purpose-run hospices for their final weeks. The hallmarks are quiet, calm, efficient pain relief, a high staff to patient ratio, and easy access and support for relatives. There is usually a religious bias, although no one is compelled to take part in the prayers.

BEREAVEMENT

One person's death is another's bereavement, and in many cases mourning begins when the approach of death is recognised. Bereavement like dying progresses through several stages and may be complicated or unusually severe. At St Christopher's Hospice in London, a predictive questionnaire has been given to the patient's relatives during the past decade to identify those likely to require special help. Negative factors are:

(a) paucity of family, social or occupational support;
(b) sudden, unexpected bereavement;
(c) ambivalent relationship with the patient, involving anger or guilt;
(d) clinging and dependency on either patient's or relative's part;
(e) poor health;
(f) other losses and upsets.

Murray Parkes (1982) has said:

it would seem that professional services and professionally supported voluntary and self-help services are capable of reducing the risk of psychiatric and psychosomatic disorders, resulting from bereavement. If help can be provided before as well as after bereavement the chances of success may be further improved.

Bereavement means loss — of an important other, of role and of acceptability, especially for women, and a change in financial status and perhaps of home.

Bereavement is met by a sense of numbness, allowing time for some internal readjustment. This is adaptive initially, but inhibiting to progress if it lasts two weeks or more. The bereaved person may say that he cannot 'take it in'. His mouth is dry and although plenty to drink is welcome, he can scarcely swallow food. The stage of acute realisation brings an urge to cry out loud. This subsides but acute pangs of grief come and go. There is an impulse to search for what has been lost in photographs, clothes, familiar places, bringing small hope and then greater disappointment. A 'sense of presence' of the dead person may be felt, or even a hallucination of him: comforting rather than alarming. Fleeting misinterpretations of sounds and sights are common in early bereavement. A little later, phrases and mannerisms characteristic of the dead person may be adopted, and, morbidly, his symptoms (Parkes, 1972).

However devotedly a bereaved person had cared for the patient, his death will release a load of guilt. Even to have harboured a negative thought is enough to cause torments of self-blame. It is understandable that such dysphoric feelings should sometimes be dealt with by displacement or suppression. Blame may be displaced to God, the family, or the doctors; suppression may lead to depression or physical symptoms.

The tasks of bereavement are: recognition of the loss; grieving; loosening the emotional ties to the dead person; and reorganisation of life. When a patient has died in hospital, the professionals involved should continue contact with the relatives for a short period, then transfer them to some other system for support, separate from the hospital itself. The first duty to a bereaved person is to provide company, to help him to realise what has happened, and to facilitate the expression of feeling: sorrow, anger or anxiety. Tears are beneficial, since it is inhibited or suppressed grief that leads to later psychiatric or physical morbidity. The terminal-care team should not be too long involved with the grieving person, whose major need is to look forward and to make adjustments for a different life. The particular situation of stillbirth has been dealt with in Chapter 8.

REFERENCES

Davidson, K. (1981) 'Toxic Psychosis', *British Journal of Hospital Medicine*, *26*, 530-7

Flynn, A. and Stewart, D. (1979) 'Where Do Cancer Patients Die? A Review of Cancer Deaths in Cuyahoga County, Ohio, 1957-1974', *Journal of Community Health*, *5*, 126-30

Hinton, J. (1972) 'Psychiatric Consultation in Fatal Illness', *Proceedings of the Royal Society of Medicine*, *65*, 1035-40

Hinton, J. (1976) 'Approaching Death', in Hill, O.W. (Ed.) *Modern Trends in Psychosomatic Medicine — 3*, Butterworth, London

Hinton, J. (1980) 'Whom Do Dying Patients Tell?', *British Medical Journal*,

281, 1328-30

Kubler-Ross, E. (1970) *On Death and Dying*, Macmillan, London

Levy, S.M. (1983) 'The Process of Death and Dying: Behavioural and Social Factors', in Burish, T.G. and Bradley, L.A. (Eds) *Coping with Chronic Disease*, Academic Press, New York

Parkes, C.M. (1972) *Bereavement: Studies of Grief in Adult Life*, Tavistock, London/Methuen, New York

Parkes, C.M. (1982) Chapter 14 in Parkes, C.M. and Stevenson-Hinde, J. (Eds) *The Place of Attachment in Human Behaviour*, Tavistock, London/Methuen, New York

Pattison, E.M. (1977) *The Experience of Dying*, Prentice-Hall, London

Petrich, J. and Holmes, T.H., (1980) Chapter 11 in Hall, R.C.W. (Ed.) *Psychiatric Presentations of Medical Illness*, Spectrum, New York

Redd, W. (1982) 'Treatment of Excessive Crying in a Terminal Cancer Patient: a Time Series Analysis', *Journal of Behavioural Medicine, 5*, 225-35

Saunders, C. (1966-7) 'The Management of Terminal Illness — 1, — 2, — 3', *Hospital Medicine 1*, 225-8; 317-20; 433-6

Selby, P. (1985) 'Measurement of the Quality of Life after Cancer Treatment', *British Journal of Hospital Medicine, 33*, 266-71

Shneidman, E. (1978) 'Some Aspects of Psychotherapy with Dying Persons', in Garfield, E. (Ed.) *Psychosocial Care of the Dying Patient*, McGraw-Hill, New York

Sobel, H. (1981) 'Towards a Behavioural Thanatology in Clinical Care', in Sobel, H. (Ed.) *Behavioural Therapy in Terminal Care: a Humanistic Approach*, Ballinger, Cambridge, Mass.

Steadford, A. (1984) *Facing Death*, Heinemann, London

15

Pharmacology in Liaison Psychiatry: Summary of General Principles

An essential factor in the assessment of a patient is what drugs he may have taken: socially, illegally, over the counter, or prescribed. Interactions between them are also of crucial importance. Perusal of current and recent drug charts and meticulous enquiry of the patient frequently provide the explanation for puzzling symptoms.

ALCOHOL

The influence of alcohol is more pervasive and far-reaching than of any other substance ingested. Since the patient may omit to mention or deliberately conceal his drinking history, a high index of suspicion is necessary in disorders which could have an ethanolic connection. In a general medical unit in London 27 per cent of admissions were attributed to alcohol use, although less than half had obvious alcohol-related disorders (Lockhart *et al.*, 1986).

Acute alcoholic intoxication

This seldom provides problems for the liaison psychiatrist. The picture varies according to dosage and individual tolerance. In the early stages depression of the reticular formation releases the cerebral neurones, with subjective exhilaration and either friendly or aggressive excitement. Underlying resentments may be revealed in paranoia, or sadness in maudlin weeping. *Manie à potu* is an acute paranoid alcoholic state of psychotic intensity, said to be due to rare sensitivity. Psychological and motor efficiency is progressively impaired in acute intoxication, resulting in ataxia, dysarthria, muddled thinking and finally drowsiness and coma. Slow stertorous breathing, subnormal temperature and muted reflexes are characteristic: the pupils may be dilated or contracted.

An upgoing plantar reflex is an alarm signal in an unconscious patient who smells of alcohol. Head injury, subdural haematoma, subarachnoid or other stroke, hypoglycaemia, bleeding from oesophageal varices and postictal state all need consideration before dismissing the diagnosis as 'drunk'. Even in the latter case respiratory depression is dangerous.

Alcoholic 'blackout' is a dose-related delayed effect of acute excessive alcohol intake (see Chapter 5). It refers to a blank in memory, not of consciousness.

Hypoglycaemia as an acute and recurrent effect of a large intake comes on six to 36 hours later. It may prove fatal if the patient falls asleep on an empty stomach and is undisturbed. Obviously the risks are considerable for a diabetic on insulin. (See Chapter 9.)

Chronic alcoholic excess

With or without a history of drunkenness this may damage virtually any organ, but the nervous and gastrointestinal systems are particularly vulnerable. The liaison psychiatrist must always be alert to the possibility that alcohol is partly or wholly responsible for a patient's symptoms (Catalan *et al.*, 1985). Essential screening includes transaminase (ALT and AST) and gamma-glutamyltransferase (GTT) tests of liver function, and assessment of mean corpuscular volume (MCV) of the red blood cells, which are enlarged in alcoholism.

Central nervous system, including psychological, presentations

Withdrawal symptoms ranging from tremor, nightmares, nausea or a fit, to full delirium tremens, may cause diagnostic anxiety if they reveal themselves unexpectedly after surgery and postanaesthatic problems are suspected. In pneumonia, delirium developing over 24-72 hours may be due in part to alcohol withdrawal (see Chapters 3 and 5). Wernicke's encephalopathy, Korsakov's psychosis, and alcoholic dementia have been discussed in Chapter 5.

Cerebellar degeneration may not always be recognised as alcoholic in origin. It usually manifests in a wide-based stance and ataxic gait. The arms are less affected, but nystagmus and dysarthria may be noticeable. Improvement is slow after stopping further alcohol intake, and giving B group vitamins parenterally and then orally for several months. Thiamine alone may be given at 10-100 mg daily by either route.

Alcoholic hallucinosis: some psychiatrists include under this heading the visual, tactile and auditory hallucinations of a withdrawal state. Others, including myself, prefer to restrict the use of the term to a hallucinatory state, usually auditory, which occurs during continued alcohol intake. It may begin with misinterpretation of the sound of a radio, the buzz of conversation in a bar, or an overheard, unrelated conversation. The condition usually subsides after three or four weeks free from alcohol but covered by major and minor tranquillisers, or may continue and come to resemble paranoid schizophrenia. A few months on, say, trifluoperazine (5-30 mg daily) may suffice to restore the patient's perceptions to normal, so long as he does not drink or unless a chronic disorder develops.

Morbid jealousy is a nearly or frankly delusional state not uncommon in alcoholics, and is similar to alcoholic hallucinosis in its psychotic nature and sometimes associated with it.

Depression of a neurotic type is commonly induced or made worse by the depressant influence of alcohol. Assessment and treatment of the depression should be delayed until the toxic effects of alcohol have subsided: about two weeks. Manic depressive patients may drink excessively in either phase of their illness, making matters worse but not altering the character of the psychosis.

Trimipramine, which is particularly sedating and does not suppress REM sleep, is generally helpful to the neurotic depressive state of a dry alcoholic.

Chronic tension and anxiety states often underlie alcohol abuse, and again, when the patient is clear of the direct effects of alcohol, the psychiatric disorder should receive attention. Hypnotics are often necessary to give the patient enough peace and rest to function without alcohol. Daytime benzodiazepines should be avoided. Chlormethiazole, even more addictive, should not be given day or night after a nine-day withdrawal period, if it is used. Tranylcypromine (10-40 mg divided) or phenelzine (30-60 mg divided) are often effective in reducing the non-drinking alcoholic's propensity to panic, but MAOIs are contraindicated in a situation of continuing drinking.

Disulfiram helps the cautious or obsessional patient particularly to resist the impulse to drink, and is used as an optional form of management for those convicted of alcohol-related offences (Brewer and Smith, 1983). For most patients the most effective method is administration of the medication, dissolved in water, by a relative or other reliable collaborator. Dosage ranges from 200-600 mg daily: it is unecessary to divide the dosage. If no-one can give the patient the medication on a daily basis it can be effective given three or four times weekly in 600 mg doses. Disulfiram implants (not available in the US) are pharmacologically unreliable but extremely effective in some patients. Implantation of inert silastine is practised by some therapists, with misinformation to the patient to induce him to believe he has had a disulfiram implant. In my view this is dishonest and likely to lead to accidents to patients who have functioning — albeit irregularly — implants, as the word gets round that implants are inactive.

Whatever drug manoeuvres are employed, the alcoholic patient requires long-continued psychotherapeutic support: individual, group or both. Alcoholics Anonymous has provided a new way of life for many alcoholics, but suits only certain personalities. The disapproval of drug treatment whether disulfiram, or antidepressant, antipsychotic, or antitension medication for underlying psychiatric disorder, by several valuable non-professional helping agencies is a grave disadvantage. The most important element in the management of alcoholic patients is persistence and readiness to start afresh many times. Help and support for the relatives of alcoholics is also necessary; the Al-Anon section of Alcoholics Anonymous offers such a service.

Peripheral nervous system

Peripheral neuropathies involve reflexes and sensation, most frequently affecting the lower limbs. A feeling like walking on cotton wool is common, or a burning sensation in the feet, especially at night. Although thiamine deficiency is thought to be implicated large oral or parenteral doses of B complex vitamins often produce disappointing results. (See *Cerebellar degeneration* above for dosage.)

Amblyopia is unusual with ethyl as opposed to methyl alcohol, which has a direct neurotoxic effect. Dimness of central vision especially affecting red and green may progress to blindness. Peripheral neuropathy is usually present, and deficiency of thiamine and hydroxocobalamin is thought to be involved. These vitamins should be given at first parenterally: thiamine 100 mg daily, hydroxocobalamin (cyanocobalamin in the US) 1 mg daily.

Gastrointestinal system

Morning nausea and vomiting may progress to chronic gastritis and ulceration. Somewhat less often, chronic diarrhoea is the presenting symptom of regular, substantial alcohol intake, particularly of red wines. Oesophagitis from the searing effect of alcohol on the mucosa causes chest discomfort, but far more serious are oesophageal varices resulting from back pressure from a cirrhosing liver. They too cause discomfort and a feeling of fulness in the chest after food, but carry the ever-present peril of a sudden disastrous bleed.

Alcohol metabolism may monopolise almost the entire supply of oxidised enzymatic co-factors in the liver and interfere competitively with most other hepatic functions. Impaired fat metabolism leads to fatty deposits, with hepatomegaly and obesity. Tender, enlarged liver — hepatitis — and at a later stage cirrhosis are well recognised results of chronic alcoholism (see Chapter 7). Hepatic encephalopathy may be acute or chronically fluctuant with impairment of mood, personality and intellect with dysarthria, ataxia and tremor. Coma and death or moderate recovery may ensure (see Chapter 3).

Chronic alcoholic pancreatitis may cause diagnostic difficulty, presenting with deep, persistent abdominal pain, and weight loss but little to show, unless episodes of acute pancreatitis supervene. Diabetes mellitus results from pancreatitis in some cases The psychiatrist may help to uncover the aetiology in such alcohol-related disorders but treatment is urgently medical initially.

Other presentations

Excessive production of mucus in the respiratory system may add to the morning hawking and retching, injected watery eyes and thick voice of the chronic imbiber. Bronchitis and pneumonia are common in alcoholics, and in the deteriorated pulmonary tuberculosis is comparatively prevalent.

Myopathies affect most obviously the limbs, and the muscles are painful, tender, weak and wasted. Cardiomyopathy may present similarly to myocardial infarction, but electrocardiographically and pathologically resembles the cardiac effects of beriberi. An increased liability to cancer of the upper gastrointestinal tract, liver and larynx should be borne in mind when dealing with a heavy drinker who is depressed, generally unwell and losing weight.

Interactions between alcohol and other drugs

In casual, social, regular or excessive use, alcohol has a potential for interaction with commonly used drugs, of which the liaison psychiatrist must be aware. Most such interactions are additive, comprising mutual enhancement of, for instance, sedative effects. Others are pharmacokinetic, arising from the particular mode of metabolism of alcohol in the liver: by alcohol dehydrogenase, the microsomal oxidising system and — for 2 per cent — by catalase. In the ordinary way alcohol is degraded to acetaldehyde, which in turn is rapidly converted to acetic acid, a rather poor energy source.

When an inexperienced drinker's liver is presented with an acute load of alcohol, mono-oxygenase enzymes may have to be used to assist alcohol dehydrogenase resulting in less efficient metabolism of certain other drugs. This means that an overdose of say, amitriptyline is far more dangerous if a social or occasional drinker helps it down with alcohol; and side-effects are commoner even with therapeutic doses.

Tolerance to alcohol develops rapidly at both cellular and metabolic levels. The former is obvious in the short-term. The degree of intoxication observed and experienced at a particular blood level is greater at the beginning than the end of a bout, since by then the cells are already accustomed to alcohol. At cellular level alcohol has a variable influence on the turnover of dopamine and noradrenaline, producing unpredictable behavioural changes. It also has a direct effect on the lipid structure of neuronal membranes, modifying the transmission of impulses in a manner comparable to numerous anaesthetic agents, and possibly interfering with their action (McInnes, 1985).

The microsomal oxidising system is particularly susceptible to induction by alcohol and other sedating drugs such as phenobarbitone, with cross-tolerance. In deliberate overdosage with anticonvulsants, tricyclic antidepressants or hypnotics, the established alcohol user may recover more quickly than a non-drinker. The induction of hepatic microsomal enzymes subsides only after weeks or months free of alcohol.

In advanced alcoholism when the liver cannot cope with even small amounts of alcohol, it is equally unable to detoxify other drugs and deal with the body's internal metabolic demands.

CNS depressants

Drugs implicated include hypnotics, sedatives, anxiolytics, neuroleptics, antidepressants, antihistamines, anticonvulsants and narcotic analgesics, including codeine. Though an additive pharmacodynamic interaction is usual, in the case of diazepam the result is synergistic and more dangerous. Particular care is necessary with long-acting benzodiazepines since the patient may not realise the drug is still active when he drinks the next day. Sedation and impaired psychomotor and cognitive functions result. Many over-the-counter medicines for coughs and colds have CNS-depressant effects.

Incidentally, the CNS-depressant action of alcohol is not ameliorated by the traditional caffeine-containing drinks such as black coffee.

Anticonvulsants

Patients on anticonvulsants should avoid alcohol. It is mildly epileptogenic in its own right, and more so in withdrawal, and because of its enzyme-inducing effects will reduce the efficacy of a steady dose of anticonvulsants.

Anti-alcoholics

Disulfiram and also citrated calcium carbimide interact with alcohol to produce unpleasant effects: flushing, headache, nausea and vomiting, palpitations, hypotension and — rarely — cardiovascular collapse. Disulfiram inhibits acetaldehyde dehydrogenase, allowing a build-up of acetaldehyde which is largely responsible for the symptoms. The 'disulfiram reaction' may also be induced accidentally if alcohol is taken with some cephalosporins, metronidazole, procarbazine and sulphonylurea antidiabetics such as chlorpropamide and tolbutamide.

Antidiabetics

Apart from this reaction in some patients there may be other undesirable interactions with alcohol. Alcohol itself stimulates insulin release, and dangerous hypoglycaemia may occur in a patient already taking antidiabetic therapy (see above). Acute ingestion of alcohol inhibits the metabolism of both the old and newer sulphonylureas, thus prolonging their action. Lactic acidosis is more likely to develop with metformin if alcohol is taken.

Antihypertensives, antianginal drugs and peripheral vasodilators

An acute load of alcohol increases the effect of all these drugs since it is a vasodilator also. Postural hypotension and syncope may result.

Oral anticoagulants

Acute alcohol intake inhibits the metabolism of coumarin anticoagulants but in chronic alcoholism enzyme induction leads to enhanced metabolism, and higher doses of anticoagulant are required. If alcohol is then withdrawn, bleeding may occur.

Non-steroidal anti-inflammatory drugs

Some of these may be obtained over the counter. There is an increased risk of gastrointestinal bleeding if they, or aspirin, are taken with alcohol.

Paracetamol

Hepatic necrosis after overdosage is caused by a specific metabolite, produced more freely in chronic alcohol users.

Narcotic analgesics

These interact with alcohol to increase respiratory depression. Self-poisoning with analgesics containing dextropropoxyphene, e.g. co-praxamol, Distalgesic, is fatal in many cases if combined with alcohol. Hepatic encephalopathy may be precipitated by sedatives, narcotic analgesics, hypokalaemia for any reason, and constipation. Diuretics given in hepatic failure may induce hypokalaemia unless potassium supplements are given (Griffin and D'Arcy, 1979; *British National Formulary*, 1985)

DRUGS ASSOCIATED WITH DEPRESSION

A frequent reason for a liaison request is because the patient appears depressed or withdrawn. Chronic or painful illness and a poor response to treatment may directly cause fatigue, anorexia or disturbed sleep and understandable disappointment, sadness and diminishing hope. Nevertheless it is well worth while to consider whether such symptoms are at least in part a drug effect. Many preparations used in general medicine have the potential for bringing on clinical depression.

Psychotropics

Benzodiazepines are used freely in general and hospital practice for hypnosis, to quell anxiety, to relax musculature or in the management of migraine. All except alprazolam are depressants, ultimately leading to retardation and tearfulness. Non-benzodiazepine sedatives and hypnotics, such as barbiturates, chloral and chlormethiazole, act similarly.

Butyrophenones, particularly benperidol, phenothiazines and other neuroleptics may produce parkinsonian symptoms and a dampening down of psychological energy. They do not cause depression in schizophrenics but may do so when used to control nausea or dizziness, or for general sedation.

Antihypertensives

Hypertension itself may be associated with depression, and paradoxically reduction of a chronically raised blood pressure may leave the patient feeling oddly deflated and down. However, hypotensive medication may have directly depressant effects. Reserpine reduces the availability of serotonin and noradrenaline centrally, potentiates acetylcholine, increases prolactin production and leads to electrolyte changes. It is well known to precipitate severe depression in those predisposed. Methyldopa reduces the activity of dopamine and noradrenaline and freely traverses the blood/brain barrier. Even in the absence of a constitutional tendency, it may lead to symptoms of endogenous depression with suicidal ideation. Clonidine, also centrally acting, may aggravate a depressive diathesis and cause insomnia, but far less frequently and less severely than methyldopa. It is used for migraine and menopausal flushes as well as in hypertension.

Peripheral alpha-blockers guanethidine and bethanidine lead to salt and water retention as with reserpine, and act on catecholamines at the synapse. They do not penetrate the blood/brain barrier to any extent but are not infrequently associated with weakness, fatigue and frank depression. Tricyclic antidepressants reduce the effectiveness of these drugs. Beta-blockers may also induce depression in up to 6 per cent of patients, but this effect is minimal with labetalol and atenolol. Propranolol may be associated with hallucinations as well as depression. A previous history does not make depression more likely if the patient takes a beta-blocker.

Steroids and some other hormones

Affective disorders, most frequently atypical depressive psychoses, occur in up to 24 per cent of patients taking adrenocorticotrophic hormone or corticosteroids — as for rheumatoid arthritis, regional ileitis, multiple sclerosis, asthma, systemic lupus erythematosus and malignant disease. Some patients become euphoric or paranoid rather than depressive: the psychosis may develop during treatment or if the medication is discontinued abruptly. Oestrogens and progestogens, whether given singly for prostatic carcinoma or male sexual deviance, or in combination in an oral contraceptive, are variably associated with depression. Private and personal attitudes and expectations concerning sexual activity are of profound importance to mood, and the taking of medication may conveniently be blamed for unhappiness.

Neurological drugs

Anticonvulsants including phenobarbitone, phenytoin, carbamazepine and ethosuximide are all depressant. The first two behave in much the same manner as alcohol and similarly are often involved in overdosage. Baclofen, a muscle relaxant, tetrabenazine used in Huntington's chorea, and levodopa and amantidine for Parkinson's disease may all lead to depression. Tetrabenazine depletes both indoleamines and catecholamines. Levodopa is associated with depression in 4 per cent of those taking it, and 1.5 per cent become manic. Bromocriptine, used in Parkinson's disease, acromegaly and pituitary-caused amenorrhoea, may set off any type of psychosis — including depressive — in the vulnerable. Selegiline (L-deprenyl), which is mainly used as an adjunct to levodopa, is an MAO-B inhibitor and is metabolised to methylamphetamine and amphetamine; it may cause euphoria or psychosis.

Narcotic analgesics and anti-inflammatory drugs

Narcotic analgesics, despite their addictive potential, may cause, among various psychiatric upsets, depression. Some patients would rather endure pain than suffer the clouding of thought and dulling of mood produced in them by opiates. Non-steroidal anti-inflammatory drugs include indomethacin, ibuprofen, piroxicam and naproxen. The first is associated with depression in about 6 per cent of cases but the incidence is somewhat less with the others, although there are other important side-effects, particularly gastrointestinal, with all (Whitlock, 1982a).

Antineoplastics

Antineoplastics such as trimethoprim, bleomycin, vincristine and cis-platinum are likely to be associated with depression. This is separate from and unconnected with the nausea and fatigue accompanying the course of treatment and the emotional effects of hair loss added to the loss of health and energy.

Antibiotics and similar drugs

Most of these can cause depression in a minority of cases who cannot be predicted. Penicillins, cycloserine, ethionamide, griseofulvin, streptomycin, tetracycline, sulphonamides, metronidazole, nalidixic acid and nitrofurantoin are among those recorded as potentially depressant.

Other unrelated drugs sometimes associated with depression include digoxin, cimetidine, cyproheptadine, choline, disulfiram, mebeverine, domperidone, pizotifen, salbutamol and — when withdrawn — appetite suppressants (Crowder and Pate, 1980).

DRUGS ASSOCIATED WITH MANIC SYMPTOMS

Manic reactions are well documented following major surgery, perhaps partly an anaesthetic/analgesic effect; after childbirth; in cerebral tumour; during haemodialysis; and after the administration of ECT and certain drugs (Whitlock, 1982b). Obviously in a patient who has had previous manic episodes any of these organic events may act as a precipitant, but in some cases there is no indication of a predisposition. Medication implicated includes antidepressants, especially clomipramine or tranylcypromine, isoniazid, corticosteroids, procarbazine, levodopa, or thyroxine given in too large an initial dosage for hypothyroidism (Josephson and Mackenzie, 1980). Amphetamines and appetite suppressants may induce a general speeding up and stimulation of mood temporarily, sometimes running into a paranoid psychosis which takes one to two weeks to subside.

Other cases involve euphoria of an organic type rather than psychosis in clear consciousness characterising mania (Cutting, 1980). The jolly disinhibition of the frontal lobe syndrome that can readily become aggressive, the fatuous euphoria of Pick's disease and sometimes multiple sclerosis, or the excitement and recklessness which may be associated with hypoglycaemia — however caused — need considering in differential diagnosis. Elation with a subjective sense of wittiness (banality to the observer) embedded in a dream-like state with altered perceptions may result from cannabis use. The mood may switch from ecstasy to terror with hallucinations and disturbed body image, and the conjunctivae are pink (Ghodse, 1983). Narcotics may produce euphoria and a sense of mental detachment as well as nausea and respiratory depression. Antidiarrhoeals and antitussives such as codeine linctus may be used in gross excess to invoke similar feelings.

Elation, garrulousness and irritability are typical of chronic intoxation with barbiturates, anticonvulsants or very large regular doses of benzodiazepines. One patient took 40 mg nitrazepam four to six times daily, obtaining supplies easily for 'so harmless a drug'. Fleeting disturbances in orientation and conscious awareness distinguish these organic states from affective disorder (Tyrer, 1980).

ORGANIC BRAIN SYNDROMES DUE TO DRUGS

Toxicity results from acute or chronic overdosage of any drug, whether taken accidentally or deliberately or mistakenly prescribed. Particular caution is needed in the over-60s, those with impaired liver function and heavy drinkers (Lishman, 1978).

Acute states

Acute states involving delirium or sometimes fits may be induced by: lithium, at serum levels over 1.3 mmol/1 for instance after taking a thiazide diuretic or if there is haemoconcentration from any cause; antiparkinsonian medication of whichever type, old or newer; corticosteroids; antidepressants including MAOIs; ergot preparations for migraine; salicylates; ephedrine and related drugs; and in the idiosyncratically susceptible chloral, chlormethiazole or cannabis.

Similar symptoms may follow sudden accidental or intended withdrawal from barbiturates, high-dose benzodiazepines, meprobamate, methaqualone or alcohol.

Chronic states

Chronic minor analgesic abuse may be suspected from tremor, ataxia, tinnitus, hyperventilation and such psychiatric effects as impaired memory, paranoia and visual hallucinations. The latter are most prevalent with pentazocine. Chronic cannabis intoxication may present a similar picture or there may be progressive personality and intellectual deterioration, as in schizophrenia. Chronic barbiturate intoxication has already been discussed aove. Anticonvulsants, with the exception of carbamazepine, may have much the same effects even at blood levels within the therapeutic range. There may be difficulties with memory, immediate and delayed, with decision making, with drive and with sociability. Children may show a fall-off of between ten and 40 points on intellectual testing over a year.

Cold remedies usually contain sympathomimetic decongestants: phenylamines such as ephedrine and phenylpropanolamine, usually taken orally, and imidazolines usually applied to the nasal mucosa. Because of their stimulant action they have an addictive potential, but may produce undesirable effects with a few days' normal use. Phenylpropanolamine is also used as an appetite suppressant in the USA, and this class of drugs has a reputation for aiding weight loss by speeding the metabolism. Phenylamines may induce hypertension, palpitations, insomnia, anxiety, visual and auditory hallucinations and paranoid fears. Imidazoline drops or sprays inevitably cause rebound nasal congestion; they may also bring on bradycardia, arrhythmias, changes in blood pressure up or down, and the same nervous effects as phenylamines. Haloperidol is the drug of choice for these symptoms (Chaplin, 1984).

Drugs of addiction

Drugs of addiction are by definition used chronically. Barbiturates, amphetamines and like stimulants have been considered. Opiates, cocaine and (although it is not strictly addictive) lysergic acid will be reviewed briefly; cannabis has been discussed already.

Heroin is the opiate most commonly used for pleasure. The psychiatrist may be asked to advise on the management of a patient claiming to be a regular user. A registered addict in the UK presents no problem. Others tend to give exaggerated estimates of their intake. When a patient is admitted as a matter of urgency for medical or surgical reasons, it is neither appropriate nor feasible to assess accurately his heroin habit. Withdrawal symptoms are evident six to 12 hours after the last dose and comprise restlessness and anxiety, sweating, yawning, lachrymation, rhinorrhoea, gooseflesh, diarrhoea and vomiting. The blood pressure rises. Chlorpromazine (25-100 mg by any route) may be used to control the symptoms or the effect of methadone, 10 mg as linctus, observed and repeated as necessary.

Cocaine is a central nervous system stimulant like amphetamine but more powerful, producing alertness, energy and confidence.

Huge doses are consumed by regular users, and a sign of its inhalation is ulceration of the nasal mucosa. It can produce a toxic psychosis of which tactile hallucinations — 'cocaine bugs' — are characteristic. Chlorpromazine ameliorates the acute state.

Lysergic acid diethylamide reached a peak of popularity in the 1960s. Its somatic effects are unimportant, deriving from mild autonomic stimulation. The psychological 'trip' lasts about six hours and consists largely of perceptual changes in all modalities and altered awareness of self. These experiences are usually quietly preoccupying but are occasionally accompanied by acute panic; the patient may plunge into danger in trying to escape. Flashbacks may recur up to two months later but are usually transient. Psilocybin, mescaline and other hallucinogens have similar but less potent effects. Neuroleptics are helpful in the acute stages (Shaw *et al.*, 1982).

Other medications which may be significant in liaison assessment include the potassium-sparing diuretics triamterene and amiloride, which sometimes cause mental confusion. Other diuretics are less likely to cause psychological disturbance unless there is hypokalaemia. Amiodarone, used in cardiac arrhythmia, may precipitate either hypo- or hyperthyroidism by releasing iodine. Antacids, used overgenerously, disturb plasma levels of sodium and magnesium with resultant mental symptoms, and prevent the absorption of cimetidine, chlorpromazine and antibiotics.

DISORDERS OF FLUID AND ELECTROLYTE BALANCE

These may occur as a result of disease, or of treatment. It is imperative that they be recognised and corrected promptly (Webb and Gehi, 1980).

Dehydration

Dehydration causes the patient to look grey and ill; his mouth is dry. Plasma levels of sodium, chloride and urea rise, and the brain is depleted of fluid. Mental confusion runs into delirium then coma. The elderly are at particular risk because of their diminished capacity to reabsorb fluid through the renal tubules. Dehydration may develop when a patient is too ill or too out of touch to respond to his thirst mechanism, or he may refuse to eat or drink because of a depressive or schizophrenic psychosis, or rarely with severe anorexia nervosa.

Loss of fluid by diarrhoea or vomiting is, of course, obvious. Restoration of fluid by mouth or 5 per cent dextrose infusion is urgent, as is treatment of the cause, with ECT in psychiatric cases.

Water intoxication

This manifests in headache, anorexia and nausea, vomiting, lassitude and later delirium, cramps, fits and finally coma. The causes are excessive intravenous infusions; or excessive oral intake of fluids with or without renal failure; inappropriate secretion of antidiuretic hormone (ADH); or certain psychiatric disorders. ADH overproduction is associated with oatcell bronchial carcinoma and central nervous system neoplasia, intermittent porphyria and some cases of schizophrenia. It may also be induced by the administration of amitriptyline, fluphenazine, chlorpromazine and thiothixene; these also encourage fluid intake by their side-effect of dry mouth. Even without psychotropic medication, personality-disordered patients with hysterical traits and schizophrenics may drink compulsively. Obviously dextrose infusions must be withheld, and the ADH antagonist demeclocycline may be tried (Ferrier, 1985).

Hyponatraemia

Hyponatraemia may result from dilution of body fluids in water intoxication or more commonly in congestive cardiac failure, cirrhosis, excessive sweating, diuresis, and Addison's disease. Indications are depression and anxiety, agnosia, muscular weakness, fatigue, hypotension, cramps, vomiting and later an acute organic brain syndrome. In liaison practice, hyponatraemia is particularly likely in oncology patients. Treatment is salt by mouth or infusion.

Hypokalaemia

Vomiting, laxative abuse, overuse of diuretics (often for slimming), or dietary deficiency as in severe anorexia nervosa, liquorice extract for ulcers or as sweets, corticosteroids, acetylsalicylic acid and penicillin may all induce hypokalaemia. Symptoms of anxiety and of muscular weakness such as backache occur, and there are characteristic electrocardiographic changes: small T, prolonged Q-T and depressed ST segment. Potassium supplements are required.

Hyperkalaemia

This occurs if potassium supplements are given to excess and results in lethargy, confusion and heart block. It may occasionally arise in sufferers from anorexia or bulimia nervosa drinking large amounts of low-calorie mineral waters and soft drinks.

Hypercalcaemia

Hypercalcaemia may follow too much vitamin D and too much milk and alkali and occurs with bone metastases, Paget's disease, hyperparathyroidism or hyperthyroidism. It produces fatigue, irritability, memory impairment and headache; a diagnosis of depression may mistakenly be made. The cause requires treatment.

Caffeinism

In clinical situations alcohol and nicotine come under the spotlight but caffeine is often overlooked. It is present in significant quantities in coffee, tea, Coca Cola and the like, over-the-counter analgesics and cold remedies and chocolate, especially plain. Caffeine is absorbed within minutes from tea or coffee, crosses the placenta and is secreted in breast milk. An average strength cup of instant coffee delivers about 70 mg of caffeine. After a dose of 200-400 mg lapses of attention are less likely during, for instance night-driving; but dangerous rebound drowsiness follows if the plasma level is not maintained.

Although caffeine can have beneficial effects, a daily intake in excess of 60 mg may cause anxiety, insomnia, restlessness, tremor, diuresis, headache and palpitations. Caffeine counteracts the action of benzodiazepines and of anticonvulsants, but not of ethanol or neuroleptics. In heavy caffeine users withdrawal effects include headache, nausea and mental depression. Patients with frequent headaches often take caffeine-containing analgesics which give temporary relief but may set up a vicious circle. Caffeinism should be remembered as a possible cause for tension-type symptoms, and coffee-drinking in particular has also been linked with hypertension, myocardial infarction, peptic ulcer and urinary cancers (Kenny and Darragh, 1985).

REFERENCES

Brewer, C. and Smith, J. (1983) 'Probation-linked Supervised Disulfiram in the Treatment of Habitual Drunken Offenders; Results of a Pilot Study', *British Medical Journal, 287*, 1282-3

British National Formulary No. 9 (1985) British Medical Association and The Pharmaceutical Press, London

Catalan, R., Bathen, R. and Litvinoff, S. (1985) 'Alcohol Abuse in Patients Admitted to a General Hospital, or Continuing Detection Failure', *British Journal of Clinical and Social Psychiatry, 3*, 56-9

Chaplin, S. (1984) 'Adverse Reactions to Sympathomimetics in Cold Remedies', *Adverse Drug Reaction Bulletin, 107*, 396-9

Crowder, K. and Pate, J.K. (1980) 'A Case Report of Cimetidine-induced Depression', *American Journal of Psychiatry, 137*, 1451

Cutting, J. (1980) 'Physical Illness and Psychosis', *British Journal of Psychiatry, 136*, 109-19

Ferrier, I.N. (1985) 'Water Intoxication in Patients with Psychiatric Illness', *British Medical Journal, 291*, 1595-6

Ghodse, A.H. (1983) 'Drug Dependence and Intoxication', in Laders, M.H. (Ed.) *Mental Disorders and Somatic Illness*, Cambridge University Press, Cambridge

Griffin, J.P. and D'Arcy, P.F. (1979) *Adverse Drug Interactions*, Wright, Bristol

Josephson, A.M. and Mackenzie, T.B. (1980) 'Thyroid-induced Mania in Hypothyroid Patients', *British Journal of Psychiatry, 137*, 222-8

Kenny, M. and Darragh, A. (1985) 'Central Effects of Caffeine in Man', in Iversen, S.D. (Ed.) *Psychopharmacology: Recent Advances and Future Prospects*, Oxford University Press, Oxford and New York

Lishman, W.A. (1978) Chapters 11, 12 and 13 in *Organic Psychiatry*, Blackwell, London

Lockhart, S.P., Carter, Y.H., Staffen, A.M., Pang, K.K., McLoughlin, J. and Baron, J.H. (1986) 'Detecting Alcohol Consumption as a Cause of Emergency General Medical Admissions', *Journal of the Royal Society of Medicine, 79*, 132-6

McInnes, G.T. (1985) 'Interactions that Matter 5: Alcohol', *Prescribers' Journal, 25*, 87-90

Shaw, D.M., Kellam, A.M.P. and Mottram, R.F. (1982) Chapter 10 in *Brain Sciences in Psychiatry*, Butterworths, London

Tyrer, P. (1980) 'Dependence on Benzodiazepines', *British Journal of Psychiatry, 137*, 576-7

Webb, W.L. and Gehi, M. (1980) 'Disorders of fluid and electrolyte balance', in Hall, R.C.W. (Ed.) *Psychiatric Presentations of Physical Illness*, Spectrum, New York

Whitlock, F.A. (1982a) 'Drugs and Depression', in *Symptomatic Affective Disorders*, Academic Press, Sydney

Whitlock, F.A. (1982b) 'Mania Secondary to Disease and Drugs', in *Symptomatic Affective Disorders*, Academic Press, Sydney

16

General Strategies for the Liaison Therapist

The most far-reaching and durable benefits from liaison work lie in improved communication and enriched understanding, both within the multidisciplinary therapeutic team and between patients and professionals. Most of this is achieved on a low-key level with problems centred on persistent physical symptoms or the patient's depression. The psychiatrist can make a useful but far from dramatic contribution (Paykel and Norton, 1982).

The least common scenario, with the psychiatrist as hero of the hour, occurs when a patient in the general hospital runs out of control, threatening violence to himself or others, damaging property or putting his health in jeopardy by, for instance ripping out his venous line. Such behaviour may result from functional or organic psychosis, (including drug-induced), gross personality disorder or acute neurosis, and the psychiatrist is urgently invited. Feelings of real sympathy for a person in the grip of ungovernable emotion, and undoubtedly frightened by it, must be made clear, and confrontation must be avoided at all costs. The ideal is a calm, unthreatening approach which engages the patient's attention and interest in a one-to-one dialogue, leading to his acceptance of the sick role — and of medication. The patient's safety and that of others are the prime considerations, however, and there is no place for heroics. In an explosive situation the first essential is discreetly to arrange sufficient back-up in case it proves impossible to talk the patient down. Appropriate medication should be drawn up.

A disturbed patient may require immediate intravenous sedation. The safest choice is haloperidol 20-60 mg with procyclidine, 10 mg, to follow to avert dystonic effects. (In the US it is preferred to give hourly repeated doses of 5-10 mg until the desired effect is achieved: physical restraints may be necessary during the procedure.) Lorazepam 5-10 mg intravenously is better in cases of alcohol or barbiturate withdrawal. In any event, pulse, respiration and blood pressure should be monitored during the next two hours. The aim is to sedate the patient sufficiently to allow time to make a working diagnosis and management plan. A suicidal patient will require special nursing observation and, exceptionally, emergency ECT until transfer to a psychiatric facility is feasible.

Case: Mr Z, 67, was actively and energetically suicidal after he came round from his prostatectomy for malignancy, and he was also a heavy drinker and bronchitic. ECT reduced the suicidal risk dramatically when large doses of sedation and antidepressants could not safely be given.

Lesser degrees of disruptive behaviour — agitation, hallucinatory excitement, screaming, non-compliance, paranoid ideas and accusations, restlessness and intolerable demands — also call for acute psychiatric involvement. Effective doses of antipsychotic or other sedating medication must be given, while considering possible adverse effects on the patient's physical condition.

STAFF SUPPORT GROUPS

The major objectives of acute psychiatric intervention are to defuse a potentially dangerous situation and to give succour to the staff. A staff support group with the liaison psychiatrist as facilitator is useful in any setting but is usually recognised as time-effective in such high-technology areas as intensive therapy, coronary care and haemodialysis units, and among the less active in oncology and geriatric wards. The tasks to address include:

(a) identification and acknowledgement of negative feelings among the staff, for instance grief at a patient's death, anxiety and resentment;
(b) open expression of feelings to each other;
(c) reduction of feelings of guilt and the unrealistic belief that the staff should be omnipotent;
(d) discussion of the difficulties in caring for unconscious or other unresponsive patients who die or recover equally ungratefully and do not remember unremitting efforts on their behalf;
(e) focusing and integrating the contributions of all concerned towards the patients' welfare.

Damaging interdisciplinary doubts and divisions are lost in a sense of shared purpose. All team members come to appreciate the rainbow complexity of the interaction between genetic, environmental, emotional and physiological influences leading to malfunction. The psychiatrist gains greatly in the exchange by keeping alive his general physicianly outlook and attributes.

In general the liaisonist is involved with a particular patient and is looked to for a range of therapies somewhat different from those of his colleagues. The main planks are medication, psychotherapy and cognitive/behavioural techniques.

MEDICATION

This is the easiest and most convenient — perhaps at times too convenient — line of attack (see Iversen, 1985).

Antipsychotics

Antipsychotics (neuroleptics, major tranquillisers) are valuable in all types of psychosis with the exception of some drug withdrawal states; in paranoid, excited and agitated states; and as an adjunct in chronic pain, nausea and pruritus.

Average daily dosages:
chlorpromazine 100-1000 mg (oral administration provides only 30 per cent effective dose compared with parenteral)
thioridazine 50-600 mg (no parenteral preparation; doses above 600 mg cannot be given because of retinal effects)
trifluoperazine 5-60 mg
perphenazine 8-24 mg
haloperidol 2-200 mg (100 mg preferred in the US) (bioavailability the same for all routes)
droperidol 10-40 mg (not used in the US except for anaesthetics)

Chlorpromazine and thioridazine both have a complex metabolism involving active metabolites. This leads to a prolonged — for weeks — antipsychotic effect despite a plasma half-life of 10-20 hours. The sedating effect lasts with the latter. These two phenothiazines are particularly useful if sedation is required. Trifluoperazine and perphenazine are better if there is paranoid ideation without excitement, and it is undesirable to make the patient drowsy. Dystonic reactions and parkinsonian effects may occur with phenothiazines and butyrophenones, especially trifluoperazine and haloperidol. Procyclidine, 10 mg intramuscularly or by mouth, or orphenadrine 20 mg and 50 mg respectively, may be required up to three times a day, but some American psychiatrists prefer to use diphenhydramine, an antihistamine with anticholinergic properties. Dosage is 25-50 mg orally, twice daily, or 50 mg intramuscularly. Haloperidol, a butyrophenone, has no significantly active metabolites so its duration of effect is shorter and more predictable. It is particularly suitable in medically ill and surgical patients, for those on amphetamines, and for manics. It is also very effective in nausea and pruritus. Droperidol has an even shorter action, mainly sedating.

Antipsychotic drugs have little respiratory depressant effect and are relatively safe to give in pregnancy. However, they may reduce the effectiveness of phenytoin, antidiabetic medication, clonidine, guanethidine and methyldopa.

Antidepressants

Antidepressants all have the disadvantage of their specific effect being slower than can be accommodated by colleagues on the general site. However, patients who are clinically depressed require these drugs whichever ward they occupy. Tricyclic antidepressants are helpful in chronic pain and their antihistaminic action is marginally helpful in peptic ulceration. Amitriptyline and doxepin both have immediate sedating effects and may give the patient his first good night's sleep. They may have sympathomimetic and anticholinergic side-effects, and caution must be employed in patients with glaucoma, urinary or cardiac difficulties, or a susceptibility to functional or organic psychosis — often the elderly.

'Second-generation' antidepressants such as maprotiline, mianserin, trazodone and lofepramine are said by the manufacturers to act more rapidly, but this is not remarkable in practice. (Lofepramine is not yet available in the US.) They have fewer side-effects, but on the whole are less efficacious than the older tricyclics. Maprotiline tends to epileptogenicity, and since it has a 50-hour half-life this can cause considerable inconvenience; it may also cause a rash. Mianserin may cause drowsiness in effective dosage and more importantly is associated with blood dyscrasias; it should not be used in the elderly. Trazodone has been associated with priapism — rarely — and worsening of arrhythmia. Viloxazine can cause nausea or migraine. Two antidepressants, zimeldine and nomifensine, have been withdrawn but others are under trial.

> *Average daily dosages of antidepressants:*
> amitriptyline 50-200 mg
> doxepin 50-200 mg
> lofepramine 70-210 mg (not available in US)
> maprotiline 50-150 mg
> clomipramine 30-150 mg (not available in US)
> mianserin 30-150 mg (30 mg for the elderly)
> trazodone 50-250 mg
> viloxazine 100-300 mg
> trimipramine 25-150 mg
> imipramine 25-150 mg
> dothiepin 25-150 mg (not available in the US)
> *MAOIs*
> tranylcypromine 10-40 mg
> phenelzine 30-60 mg
> isocarboxazid 20-30 mg

Monoamine oxidase inhibitors are useful for patients with atypical depression, tension states and psychosomatic symptoms, but impose restrictions on prescribing not only during their administration but for ten days afterwards. This is generally unacceptable to other physicians except on an outpatient basis. The use of antidepressants during pregnancy is discussed in Chapter 8. The antipsychotics all have some integral anticholinergic effects at high dosage, particularly thioridazine. They comprise dry mouth, blurred vision, constipation, urinary difficulties, effects on cardiac conduction and occasionally a confusional state. Alpha-adrenergic blockade may lead to hypotension and a high resting pulse rate with neuroleptics.

Anxiolytics and hypnotics

Most inpatients sleep badly and many are anxious, so sedating medication is in universal demand. Barbiturates are effective agents but have fallen into disrepute because of their addictive potential and the fact that the dangers of overdosage and of withdrawal from them are worse than with narcotics. Since their introduction in 1961 the *benzodiazepines* have come to replace barbiturates apart from some anticonvulsant and anaesthetic use.

Benzodiazepines are usually given orally, and are absorbed slowly by this route. Those most rapidly absorbed are triazolam (a hypnotic) and alprazolam, and among those most commonly used clorazepate and diazepam. Diazepam is also particularly lipid soluble and so it enters the brain (or the foetus) rapidly compared, for instance, with chlordiazepoxide. Neither diazepam nor chlordiazepoxide is absorbed reliably if given intramuscularly, and intravenous diazepam is irritating to the venous lining unless in an emulsion. For effective parenteral administration lorazepam is the best of the benzodiazepines. It is the drug of choice in a limited course for alcohol withdrawal, it can be given by any route, and it has no adverse hepatic effect.

Lorazepam and oxazepam are particularly useful in the elderly and those with hepatic impairment since these drugs have no active metabolites and are excreted quickly and easily in the urine. Where hepatic function is compromised by whatever cause, diazepam and chlordiazepoxide among the benzodiazepines, and meprobamate, barbiturates and propranolol should be avoided. The relaxing effect of benzodiazepines, like that of alcohol, may also reduce useful inhibitions and release suppressed aggression, despair or lust. Various anecdotes have been published of exemplary characters unexpectedly beating up their wives or shoplifting after taking benzodiazepines.

Benzodiazepines reduce the time taken to fall asleep and increase the duration of stage 2 sleep. REM sleep and the deeper stages of non-REM sleep, 3 and 4, are reduced, however. Normal hypnotic doses can cause dangerous depression of the medullary respiratory centre in patients with obstructive airways disease, or cardiovascular depression in those suffering from congestive cardiac failure or hypovolaemic states. Apart from these acute risks the long-term effects of hypnotic use are uncertain. Nevertheless it is unarguable that those who complain of poor sleep do suffer and may have an increased mortality risk (Oswald, 1986). A moral stance against benzodiazepine hypnotics is unkind — and silly. While the general dosage of benzodiazepines varies widely according to the patient's level of arousal, use of alcohol or experience of benzodiazepines or barbiturates, hypnotic doses vary less.

Average hypnotic doses of benzodiazepines:
flurazepam 15-30 mg
temazepam 20-40 mg
triazolam 0.5-1.5 mg
lorazepam 1-3 mg
lormetazepam 1-3 mg (not available in US)
nitrazepam 5-15 mg (not available in the US)

Diazepam and other benzodiazepines with active metabolites may have adverse cumulative effects, so that the patient gradually slows down, learns and remembers less well, and develops a low, unconfident mood. Concurrent use of cimetidine doubles the plasma level of diazepam. Withdrawal effects including fits are likely with long-continued use of more than 10 mg lorazepam or more than 60 mg diazepam daily. None of the benzodiazepines should be used in pregnancy.

Propranolol, a beta-blocker, is sometimes used to reduce the somatic symptoms of anxiety: palpitations, tremor, sweating and dizziness. It has no sedative effect. Doses range from 40 to 240 mg daily: less than 20 mg will not reach the brain. After chronic use at therapeutic doses, withdrawal must be gradual or all the symptoms return in exaggerated form.

THERAPEUTIC MANOEUVRES NOT BASED ON MEDICATION

These comprise: psychotherapy, in its many forms; behavioural therapy, relaxation techniques, hypnotherapy and biofeedback, each of which is described later under the heading 'Behavioural Medicine' and cognitive therapy.

Psychotherapy

This term covers a range of treatments mediated by verbal exchange and aimed at relieving symptoms and improving social adjustment (Walton, 1983). The patient is helped to talk his way out of his difficulties.

Individual psychotherapy

This is the commonest type. It is part of all transactions between patient and professional, to some degree. As a formal therapy it comes in several styles, for instance analytical, supportive and expressive. Analytical psychotherapy requires more commitment from therapist and patient than is possible in liaison work, in which psychotherapy usually comprises four to six 50-minute sessions, sometimes followed by a group.

Supportive psychotherapy may be conducted by the psychiatrist himself or by another interested team member under supervision. It is appropriate in situations of stress, for instance during an exacerbation of ongoing illness, or when the diagnosis has emerged of a disease that carries a death warrant such as AIDS, or long-term threat and uncertainty, like multiple sclerosis or diabetes mellitus. It is natural to be anxious even with minor symptoms, and serious illness evokes fear, shame and impaired self-esteem (Rodin, 1984). Changes in body image are particularly upsetting whether due to the hair loss of a patient undergoing chemotherapy or the limb loss of amputee. The altered appearance of an ill person is frightening to him, as is the response of his relatives and friends. Supportive therapy seeks to ameliorate these negative emotions and to bolster adaptive coping methods. Communication itself is therapeutic especially with a receptive, professionally trained listener. Release of pent-up, worrying material — catharsis — provides some relief, as does reassurance, explicit or implicit in the therapist's continuing calm. Reassurance should not be facile, unrealistic or dismissive, but must convey that, serious though his situation may be to the patient, there are some aspects which are capable of improvement. A physically ill person may feel anger and frustration at his helplessness, and resentful of those who are well. Because of his dependency he is afraid to express his hostile feelings. It helps him to be allowed to do so in a situation in which there will be understanding and no repercussions.

Sympathy is essential at the beginning of supportive psychotherapy but must be offered increasingly sparingly, preferably when the patient has made some desirable effort. Although sympathy must not be an automatic, limitless resource, interest and concern should continue undiminished. The patient needs to feel that he is intrinsically of value, rather than being judged for his good looks, his strength or his talents. Time, that most precious commodity, spent with the patient conveys his worth better than anything else. For a patient whose self-esteem has sunk low, the load of providing time for him needs to be spread across the whole team, not just his main therapist.

Denial is a frequent reaction to an unpalatable diagnosis. Although it can lead the patient to take risks with his health, it should not lightly be broken down. It allows the patient to continue longer with something like a normal life and to gain the rewards and stimulation this brings. The therapist should not be drawn into agreeing that symptoms are of no significance, but nor need he insist on discussing the full implications until the patient clearly signals his readiness to face reality.

Many patients need supportive psychotherapy to help them through a crisis. Depressed patients should be discouraged from voluntarily giving up work: it may be a lifeline later. For those who need longer-term support, transfer to a supportive group, self-help or professionally led, is desirable.

Expressive or interpretive psychotherapy

This focuses on the patient's psychic conflicts and maladaptive responses and on ways of resolving them. In liaison work it is of particular value for patients who are judged to be using physical symptoms to avoid or conceal personality and interpersonal problems. Any insight they gain will be of benefit not only at present but also in dealing with future stress. Early experiences and relationships are explored and related to the patient's reactions in the current situation. Habitual defences are learned in childhood. In psychotherapy, maladaptive patterns are exposed and alternatives discussed.

> *Case*: Mr R. was in a competitive business. When he had his coronary thrombosis he was 58. He did not recover as quickly as anticipated and continued to complain of pain and weakness. It emerged that when Mr R. was a boy his father has sustained a back injury and remained an invalid while his mother had devoted herself to his care. Psychotherapy including his wife enabled Mr R. to recognise his maladaptive wish to repeat a family pattern and helped him to work out a reasonable rehabilitatory regimen.

Dylan Thomas, the Welsh poet who died from alcoholic excess, had been indulged by his mother all through his early years, which was her method of expressing love. In particular she spoonfed him whenever he was ill even in his 20s. When he ran into problems associated with adult responsibiilty he escaped by drinking so much that he became physically helpless and 'had to' return to his mother to be nursed. Insight-directed therapy might have been a useful approach.

Group psychotherapy

Appropriately in the context of general hospital psychiatry the originator of this treatment, Pratt (1907) was an internist in Boston. He aimed to increase the knowledge and morale of sufferers from pulmonary tuberculosis. During the last 40 years, group therapy has become widespread and varied. The types relevant to those with physical symptoms are essentially supportive. Patients with specific problems may be directed to self-help groups such as Alcoholics Anonymous, Weight Watchers or the new groups for those who have positive HIV serology: they are usually helpful on an outpatient basis. Therapist-led groups among medical and surgical inpatients are necessarily open, not closed or restricted by contract to attend. They usually comprise patients with similar physical disorders, for example asthma, postmyocardial infarction, and metastatic malignancy. They share a common loss of function, fear of death and anxiety or irritation about the response of healthy people.

The optimum number for a group is between six and twelve: if there are less than four, free expression of feelings is inhibited. Prime objectives are honesty and open discussion and through these the modification of damaging attitudes and behaviour, realisation of self-deception, and the fostering of personal development. To get some interaction going it is sometimes useful to ask each member in turn his views on a relevant subject. One issue that needs attention is the meaning of his illness to each individual, and its effect on his acceptability (Kanas and Farrell, 1984).

It is the energy generated in the patient by a modicum of fear, distress or anger that provides the fuel for change. A degree of psychological upset is thus inevitable for the group to be effective but progress must be made at a pace which avoids disabling anxiety or social conflicts. The group leader is a catalyst, a safety valve and the illuminator of latent issues and what is common to apparently individual experiences. This tends to instil hope. Group work is particularly appropriate for patients with chronic disorders who have maladaptive relationships with family, friends or colleagues (Yalom, 1983).

Chronic symptoms: of these the most persistent and often difficult to explain organically is pain (see Chapter 4). It may derive from such diverse causes as diverticular disease, diabetes mellitus, osteoarthritis, hiatus hernia and bone cancer. Disabling pain or other symptoms may be maintained by a linking mechanism between pain, reduced activity, weakness, depression, enhanced awareness of pain and apathy. Inappropriate use of analgesia and poor compliance with medical advice are often side-effects of depression. These factors need airing in the group, as do dependency problems with chronic ill health. Physical symptoms may suit a patient's hidden neurotic needs and be welcomed, or produce bitter envy. Either way the care giver becomes the target for unreasonable demands. Relationships deteriorate unless the patient is helped towards insight, which is often easier to acquire in a group.

Self-regulation theory in chronic disease has been developed by Nerenz and Leventhal (1983). They postulate two feedback loops, one for controlling dangerous physical distress. Coping implies a flexible and adaptive style responsive to the varying demands of the disease process and to the patient's personal feelings. In an acute episode of illness a major adjustment may be made, temporarily submerging the patient's individuality. A similar attitude in chronic illness would mean that the patient would cease to exist except, for instance, as a case of cancer, as an arthritic or as a hypertensive. This is a recipe for relentless advance in symptomatology. The patient's self-esteem and feelings of worth require constant refreshment, and if he has a dip in mood this should call for special concern equally with the appearance of new organic symptoms. Within the limits of feasibility the patient should ensure that his needs for stimulus, human contact, affection, activity and relaxation are met as are those for nutrition. Group therapy can provide reminders.

Family therapy

This is obviously apposite when the invalid is a child, but is also useful in renal haemodialysis and other situations involving the family in one member's illness. General systems and cybernetics theory suggest a here-and-now interactional approach, assuming that symptoms are reinforced by interactional patterns. The aim is to alter the family's system of relating to each other.

Case: Emma, 16, was born with a mild left hemiplegia and at 15, after a fall, developed a dystonia of her left arm. Her mother was torn with guilt as the possible cause of Emma's problem and never corrected her. Her husband was content to let his wife take full responsibility for their daughter and spent more time with their son. The latter was 18, was good at sport and had several girlfriends Emma's moodiness and dystonia steadily worsened, influenced by the way her family functioned.

Minuchin *et al*. (1978) devised what they call structural therapy with the families of patients with psychosomatic disorders, particularly anorexia nervosa. Tangible goals are set, only achievable through modification of family relationships.

Couples therapy

The pair may be married, living together, heterosexual or homosexual. Physical or sexual symptoms in one partner put a strain on the relationship and may allow the emergence of neurotic reactions. The disturbances and unmet needs of early childhood are often re-enacted in a marriage. Poor self-esteem and a feeling of deprivation brought on by illness may rekindle deeply rooted emotions of a similar nature. The aim of therapy is to make overt and understandable what is covert: through exploration of each partner's childhood family relationships. The therapist must make an alliance with each of the pair, and constantly change sides in his support (Shapiro, 1984; Perris *et al.*, 1986).

Behavioural medicine

The application of the theory and methods of behavioural science to the problems of physical disorders developed in the 1970s (Pomerleau and Brady, 1979). The emphasis is on the modification of overt behaviour contributing to illness, and the application of special techniques in the management of symptoms of organic disease and unpleasant effects of some somatic treatments. Chemotherapy, for instance, often induces nausea. Techniques include: behaviour therapy, relaxation, imagery, hypnosis, autohypnosis, biofeedback and cognitive therapy.

Behaviour therapy

This embraces a bundle of techniques, some empirical, loosely aimed at improving the patient's well-being and functioning by a directed change in his behaviour (Bebbington, 1979). Maladaptive or inappropriate responses are extinguished and replaced through an individually tailored programme of negative and positive reinforcement, respectively. The rewards that act as positive reinforcers, for instance for weight gain in anorexia nervosa, are a graded series: having visitors, being allowed out of bed to bathe, getting up in the day, choosing the diet, etc. Undesirable behaviours susceptible to this method include smoking, alcoholism, counterproductive pain or illness behaviour (Sternbach, 1974; Geden *et al.*, 1984; Tyrer, 1986).

Abnormal illness behaviour

Illness behaviour comprises the patient's reactions to bodily symptoms as he perceives them. Normal and desirable illness behaviour includes anxiety, help-seeking and more or less co-operation with professional advice, followed either by restoration to health and previous activity or whatever compromise is viable. With disease seen as a major threat to life or to lifestyle there are temporary adjustment strategies: denial, regression, withdrawal, irritability. Even in the most tragic and traumatic situations most patients find a reasonable adaptation within a few months (see Chapters 12 and 14). Personal and family experience of illness, and sociocultural expectations influence the patient's pattern of response. Mechanic (1986) addresses — but does not solve — the problem of why people exposed to similar stressors respond differently. Why do women more than men react with depression, neurotic upsets, demoralisation and overdosage, or reliance on medication? Why do men tend towards drink, hard drugs and violence under stress? Why is the black population of the US low on suicide and high on homicide compared with the whites? How is it that the Chinese show the somatic manifestations of depression but not the Western-style affective change? Fashion has swept away gross hysterical symptoms and histrionics in Europe and North America, but more mundane, or subtle, somatisation of distress is commonplace, absorbing much medical care. Patients may have particular difficulty in disentangling physical and psychologically mediated symptoms in convalescence; weakness, anergy, dizziness and poor appetite may be of either type.

Probably the most important variable affecting illness behaviour is the patient's personality and especially a predisposition to introspection: the tendency to think about oneself, one's functioning and one's feelings. Attention to self increases the prevalence of reporting psychological and physical symptoms, and negative self-evaluations. By Mechanic's hypothesis, people with this orientation are more easily upset than others, seek more help, cope less well and tend to exaggerate their suffering.

It is probably among patients of this disposition that *abnormal illness behaviour* is likely to develop, and involve the liaison psychiatrist. Pilowsky (1969) defines it as:

> the persistence of a maladaptive mode of perceiving, evaluating and acting in relation to one's own state of health, despite the fact that a doctor (or other appropriate social agent) has offered a reasonably lucid explanation of the illness and the appropriate course of management to be followed.

This definition does not include psychiatric illness precipitated by the patient's predicament. Pilowsky (1978) later tried classifying the range of abnormal illness behaviours as illness-affirming, illness-denying and neuropsychiatric: with no particular clarification of the issues. The liaison psychiatrist still has the task of making a working judgement of why the patient's body/mind became destabilised at all, and why now; and what his symptoms mean to him: disaster or escape; rejection or loving care; more influence or less over important others; and what his hopes and/or expectations from medical care are.

In a situation in which the patient's illness behaviour is a handicap to him rather than a benefit (however subtle), behavioural methods of management are appropriate. They involve the whole therapeutic team and the relatives, and comprise praise and reward for normal or 'well' talk or activity, but only necessary attention served without the garnish of interest for complaint (see chapter 3).

In situations of *fear and avoidance* two behavioural approaches are in common use: slow desensitisation and flooding (Stern, 1978). The former is likely to be more appropriate in patients with physical symptoms loath to undertake therapeutic or normal activities, or refusing operation. The essentials are muscular relaxation, rapport with the therapist and a hierarchical presentation of feared situations or activities in imagination or in practice. The rate of progress is determined by the time available (e.g. before surgery) and the patient's tolerance (Wolpe, 1958).

Relaxation

This is the most basic technique in behaviour therapy. Muscular relaxation brings in its train reduction of arousal, slowing of pulse and respiration, peripheral vasodilation and lowering of the blood pressure. Training for self-induced relaxation requires daily practice for at least a fortnight so that the patient learns by repeating the process. The therapist should conduct the first one or two sessions, when the patient can continue with the use of an audiotape, preferably made by his therapist. In teaching relaxation it is not desirable to tell the patient to tense his muscles before relaxing them. Starting with the soles of his feet and working upwards he should be encouraged to induce the state of warmth and muscular relaxation felt on waking in the morning, before beginning to stir or when nearly asleep at night. Key words repeated in the therapist's soft, continuous flow — lasting ten to 15 minutes — are 'warm', 'safe', 'relaxed', 'refreshed', 'peaceful'. The patient may also like to have a word to concentrate on as he begins relaxation: for instance 'rose', 'smile', 'silk', or 'pool'.

Relaxation is an adjunct to other forms of behavioural treatment and is directly beneficial in hypertension, irritable bowel, vaginismus, organic or psychogenic pain, hyperventilation and dyspnoea. The

Eastern techniques of meditation and yoga also induce relaxation.

Imagery

This has similarities with muscular relaxation and often complements it. Relaxation deepens with imagery, and imagery can only be directed at will if the patient is relaxed. It is largely visual, but other modalities may be involved. To deepen and give a focus to relaxation I ask the patient to visualise a tropical island with sand, sky and trees, to feel the warmth on his skin and to hear the endless sound of the sea. In the Lamaze programme for natural childbirth visual imagery is used to enhance relaxation and reduce pain. Organic pain may sometimes be greatly ameliorated by concentration on an imagined sensation of warmth in the affected part. More controversial is the use of visualisation in the management of malignancy (Simonton *et al.*, 1978). Intense focusing on an image or sensation may induce physiological change. This occurs with pornography, but may be tested more acceptably by concentrating on the look, smell and sharp taste of a juicy lemon. With unwanted thoughts, as discussed under cognitive therapy, imagery may be used to interrupt them, for instance visualising a tree or a cake.

Positive imagery aims at improving the patient's situation, experiences and attitudes in a non-intrusive, unthreatening way. Regular daily periods are spent in determinedly pleasant daydreams. Guided imagery (Leuner, 1969) is a short cut to understanding the patient's inner conflicts by getting him to imagine and describe a 'waking dream' about a series of set subjects: meadow, brook, mountain, house, edge of woods, encounter with relatives, sexual attitudes, lion, ego ideal, swamp, volcano, picture book. The patient's imagery reflects his fears and feelings: it is through discussion of these that he may be helped to cope better.

Hypnosis

This is an induced altered state of consciousness enhancing suggestibility in those motivated to change. Women tend to be better subjects than men, and an IQ of more than 40 is required. Patients with clear left-brain dominance and the ability to concentrate well are susceptible to hypnosis unlike those with a right-brain bias and broadened attention (Grist, 1984). The patient must be warm and comfortable, his head must be supported, and the light must not be harsh. A blanket over the patient makes him feel cared for and dependent.

In a gentle, monotonous voice timed to the patient's breathing, the therapist suggests what is already true: that the patient is feeling warm and relaxed, that his eyelids are heavy, that his body is heavy, limp, sinking in the couch . . . Relaxation is indicated by quiet, slow, regular breathing. The patient is instructed in simple direct language what he is to do, e.g. stop smoking, with the rewards and happiness that will follow. Various symptoms such as angina, migraine or nausea may be reduced by posthypnotic suggestion. The disadvantage is that the patient really requires a course of the therapy, and time may make this impracticable (Shaw, 1977).

Autohypnosis

In this the patient is taught relaxation techniques, enhanced by imagery (see above), followed immediately by the suggestion that his mind like his muscles will relax as the therapist counts to five. The suggestions appropriate to the individual are repeated several times, and the patient is invited to open his eyes and find himself refreshed, relaxed and confident when the reverse count is made from five to one. Autohypnosis can be learned, after the first one or two sessions, from an audiotape. It is useful for asthmatics and hyperventilators, before dentistry, with gastrointestinal problems, in alcohol excess and in insomnia, and for the side-effects of cancer therapy, to name a few. It is effective only in relation to the patient's own determination to change for the better.

Biofeedback

This depends on an electronic feedback system that gives the patient immediate information on a particular aspect of his physiological status. This enables him to make a conscious effort to adjust the situation and to know at once if he is producing any change. In the early 1970s it was hailed as a panacea, but even then some experts stressed its limitations (Birk, 1973; Gaarder and Montgomery, 1981).

Areas in which biofeedback has had some success include: trauma, for instance relearning bowel control after surgery; neurological damage, for instance relearning after a stroke; stress symptoms, for instance migraine, indigestion; functional derangements, including muscle spasm, for instance in irritable bowel, oesophageal spasm and tension headache; Raynaud's syndrome; hypertension before irreversible changes have occurred; insomnia.

Cognitive therapy

This treatment approach is designed to improve the psychiatric state and also physical functioning by correcting maladaptive thinking patterns. It developed as a reaction against the mechanical manipulations of the behaviourists. Whereas other treatments in psychiatry aim at inducing changes in thoughts and mood secondarily, cognitive therapy focuses directly on the patient's way of construing his situation and experience. Beck (1963, 1964) formulated the theory that the primary disorder in depression lies in recurrent distorted and dysfunctional thinking; a similar model for anxiety has also been elaborated (Butler and Mathews, 1984).

Although we may not agree that faulty cognition is the aetiological basis of emotional disorders and their sequelae, it is not unreasonable to assume that it may help to maintain symptoms. Cognitive methods may be applied in essentially neurotic disorders: depression, anxiety, eating disorders and other harmful habits and psychosomatic symptoms. It may help with worry and problems in living due to physical disease.

Up to 20 sessions are recommended by some cognitive therapists (Gelder, 1985). In liaison work between four and ten is a realistic aim. The first is devoted to explaining the treatment and helping the patient to assess his current level of functioning. He is asked to keep a diary of his activities, pain or other symptoms where appropriate, and of his mood and thoughts in reaction to these and to daily events. With the record as evidence the patient is helped to identify recurrent negative ways of thinking. These derive from the single-minded application to all that happens of an irrational, self-destructive assumption: for instance that the patient is totally unlovable and despicable, a confirmed failure in every way, or that he is doomed to a dreadful fate or disastrous loss of control. By the Socratean method of his having to answer questions the patient is guided towards considering alternative interpretations. This allows him a choice of responses rather than helpless acceptance. As well as keeping a record, between sessions the patient should have a behavioural task to perform. A change of attitude is stimulated by positive experience as well as through argument.

Cognitive restructuring for anxiety and for related symptoms or such responses as eating or drinking too much involves focusing on the sensations rather than the feared situation; and learning relaxation techniques. In eating disorder the obese and bulimia nervosa patients, similarly to depressives, indulge in automatic self-denigration which needs correction. In anorexia nervosa intrusive thoughts about weight, shape, goodness and eating require identification and change.

Other problems which may respond to a cognitive approach are those associated with disability, divorce, bereavement or redundancy: all types of loss that lower self-esteem. A general problem-solving techniques is as follows.

(1) Help the patient to define his problems clearly and subdivide them into sub-problems.
(2) Help him to consider and compare possible solutions to each.
(3) Help him to choose a particular solution and make a plan of action: to operate in defined stages.
(4) Help him to assess the results and the relative value of each tactic. Begin again at (1) if the outcome is unsatisfactory.

OTHER PROFESSIONALS

By definition liaison work depends upon contributions from other disciplines, and the treatment package upon consensus. The multidisciplinary team may include any or all of these as well as the medical input: psychologist, social worker, occupational therapist, physiotherapist, speech therapist, nursing staff.

Psychologists

Psychologists are invaluable and, depending on the local situation, may take a leading role or be scarcely available. Behavioural medicine — a modern concept — is first cousin to clinical psychology, and psychologists are usually skilled in behavioural techniques. Surgeons and physicians sometimes feel more at ease with a psychologist rather than a psychiatrist assessing and even treating their patients. Psychiatrists are associated in the minds of colleagues and their patients with serious mental disorders and mood-changing medication on the one hand, and analytical delving into family secrets on the other. Psychology holds less threat, less stigma and is often concerned with 'normal' people, for instance for vocational guidance. Psychiatric terminology may be confusing while psychological reports are more cut-and-dried. Nevertheless the best management for the patient is to have psychiatric and psychological expertise at his service. In particular the psychiatrist is needed when there are medical diagnostic complexities, and sometimes the need for psychopharmacotherapy.

Psychologists' assessments are precise and orderly, although limited to the context of their tests. Evaluation of cognitive status through the Wechsler Intelligence Scale (WAIS), the Wechsler Intelligence Scale for Children (WISC) or Raven's Progressive Matrices, properly interpreted, and specific tests (for instance for memory, visual and verbal, for perceptual difficulties and for vocabulary), may help in the localisation of brain damage. A discrepancy of more than 15 points between the verbal and performance scores of the WAIS is significant. In global fall-off or right-sided damage, verbal scores are better than performance whereas with left-sided lesions the opposite pattern predominates. Careful application of psychological tests helps to distinguish focal from general problems, and in the elderly depression from dementia (Anastasi, 1976; Vingoe, 1981).

> *Case*: Mrs Y., 70, appeared depressed and obtained a suicide kit; she had been having trouble with her memory for two years. Psychological testing revealed her to have an IQ of 116, no indications of depression but gross short-term memory impairment. Investigation uncovered the history of a fall on the ice two winters ago, and CT scanning showed abnormality in the right more than the left temporal lobe. Mrs Y was saved from treatment for depression or incarceration for dementia and she was also saved from being left to fend for herself.

Projective tests such as the Rorschach and other types may help in the diagnosis of functional psychoses, and a wide range of tests of personality and of attitudes give an indication of individual strengths and weaknesses and likely responses to stress. This may, for instance, be psychosomatic, hypochondriacal, hysterical or in the form of psychiatric symptoms, particularly anxiety and depression. The Present State Examination (Wing *et al.*, 1975) is a structured clinical interview to assess mental state and express it numerically. Although developed and used by psychiatrists, psychologists also use it as a diagnostic aid, and it is sometimes of value in liaison work.

As discussed above psychologists are skilled in the treament modalities of behavioural medicine, and the current trend is for them to undertake the psychological management (apart from medication) of increasing numbers of patients.

Social workers

Social workers play a key role in liaison work. A major proportion of self-injurers and also of those succumbing at a particular time to physical illness do so in reaction to social problems, and the illness itself may produce further such difficulties. Advice and help with the essentials of living — money, home, work and family — come from the social worker. When they have time, social workers provide excellent realistic but supportive psychotherapy, one-to-one or group.

Occupational therapists

Occupational therapists are vital in the assessment of a patient's skills in daily living, within whatever physical or psychological limitations they have. On the treatment side occupational therapy helps patients with social, vocational or simple cooking skills, encourages self-expression and boosts confidence. Future plans for a patient must often be based on advice from this discipline.

Physiotherapists

Physiotherapists are involved with many hospital patients, for example those with chest problems, and those needing mobilisation after stroke and rehabilitation of muscles and joints. It is the physiotherapist who instils hope and gives the patient a sense of progress when everything else is at a standstill. Physiotherapy inculcates a feeling of returning strength and well-being and so of increasing self-esteem.

Speech therapists

Speech therapists, more than any, help to dispel the agonising frustration of patients unable to make themselves understood because of cerebral insult or throat surgery. No function is more vital for a human than communication.

Nurses

Nurses are nearer to the patients than anyone else, sharing their lives, including the most intimate aspects, day and night. When a patient is in emotional or physical distress or has humiliating problems with bodily control or smell he can accept a nurse's help more easily than that of any other. It is a nurse whom the patient wants to see when he comes round from an anaesthetic or emerges, perplexed, from delirium. Specialist nurses give the most valuable practical help and advice with ileostomy, colostomy and home or hospital haemodialysis. It is they who make it possible for sometimes elderly and often frightened patients (and their relatives) to cope with new, strange techniques for living. Because so much of the patients' burdens are, perforce, shared with the nurses, they more than other professionals need and deserve support themselves. Particular account should be taken of nurses' opinions both because of their unrivalled inside information and to accord to this great profession the dignity it warrants.

REFERENCES

Anastasi, A. (1976) *Psychological Testing*, Macmillan, New York

Bebbington, P. (1979) 'Behaviour Therapy', in Hill, P., Murray, R. and Thorley, A. (Eds) *Essentials of Postgraduate Psychiatry*, Academic Press, London

Beck, A.T. (1963) 'Thinking and Depression: I. Idiosyncratic Content and Cognitive Distortions', *Archives of General Psychiatry, 9*, 324-33

Beck, A.T.(1964) 'Thinking and Depression: II, Theory and Therapy', *Archives of General Psychiatry, 10*, 561-71

Birk, L. (Ed.) (1973) *Biofeedback: Behavioural Medicine*, Grune & Stratton, New York

Burish, T.G. and Bradley, L.A. (Eds) (1983) Chapters 1 and 18 in *Coping with Chronic Disease*, Academic Press, New York

Butler, G. and Mathews, A. (1984) 'Cognitive Processing in Anxiety', *Advances in Behaviour Research and Therapy, 5*, 51-62

Gaarder, K.R. and Montgomery, P.S. (1981) *Clinical Biofeedback: 2, ,* Williams and Wilkins, New York

Geden, E., Beck, N. K., Hauge, G. and Pohlman, S. (1984) 'Self-report and Psychophysiological Effects of Pain-coping Strategies', *Nursing Research, 33*, 260-5

Gelder, M. (1985) 'Cognitive Therapy', in Granville-Grossman, K. (Ed.)

Recent Advances in Clinical Psychiatry — 5, Churchill Livingstone, Edinburgh

Grist, L. (1984) 'Hypnosis Depends on Left-brain Dominance', *New Scientist,* 2 August 1984, p. 36

Iversen, S.D. (Ed.) (1985) *Psychopharmacology: Recent Advances and Future Prospects,* Oxford University Press, Oxford

Kanas, N. and Farrell, D. (1984) 'Group Psychotherapy', in Goldman, H.H. (Ed.) *Reviews of General Psychiatry,* Lange, California

Leuner, H. (1969) 'Guided Affective Imagery: a Method of Intensive Psychotherapy', *American Journal of Psychotherapy, 23,* 4-14

Mechanic, D. (1986) 'The Concept of Illness Behaviour: Culture, Situation and Personal Predisposition', *Psychological Medicine 16,* 1-7

Minuchin, S., Rosman, B. and Baker, L. (1978) *Psychosomatic Families,* Harvard University Press, Harvard

Nerenz, D.R. and Leventhal, H. (1983) Chapter 2 in Burish T.G. and Bradley, L.A. (Eds) *Coping with Chronic Disease,* Academic Press, New York

Oswald, I.l (1986) 'Drugs for Poor Sleepers?' *British Medical Journal, 292,* 715

Paykel, E.S. and Norton, K.R.W. (1982) 'Masked Depression', *British Journal of Hospital Medicine, 28,* 151-7

Perris, C., Arrindell, W.A., Perris, H., Eisemann, M., van der Ende, J. and von Knorring, LK. (1986) 'Perceived Depriving Parental Rearing and Depression', *British Journal of Psychiatry, 148,* 170-5

Pilowsky, I (1969) 'Abnormal Illness Behaviour', *British Journal of Medical Psychology, 42,* 347-51

Pilowsky, I. (1978) 'A General Classification of Abnormal Illness Behaviours', *British Journal of Medical Psychology, 51,* 131-7

Pomerleau, O.F. and Brady, J.P. (Eds) (1979) *Behavioural Medicine: Theory and Practice,* Williams and Wilkins, Baltimore

Pratt, J.H. (1907) 'The Class Method of Treating Consumption in the Homes of the Poor', *Journal of the American Medical Associaton, 49,* 755-9

Rodin, G.M. (1984) 'Psychotherapy of Patients with Chronic Medical Disorders', in Goldman, H.H. (Ed) *Review of General Psychiatry,* Lange, California

Shapiro, R.J. (1984) 'Marital Therapy', in Goldman, H.H. (Ed) *Review of General Psychiatry,* Lange, California

Shaw, H. (1977) *Hypnosis in Practice,* Bailliere Tindall, London

Simonton, OI.C., Matthews-Simonton, S. and Creighton, J. (1978) *Getting Well Again,* J.P. Tarcher, New York

Stern, R. (1978) *Behavioural Techniques,* Academic Press, London

Sternbach, R.A. (1974) *Pain Patients: Traits and Treatment,* Academic Press, New York

Tyrer, S.P. (1986) 'Learned Pain Behaviour', *British Medical Journal, 292,* 1-2

Vingoe, F.J. (1981) *Clinical Psychology and Medicine,* Oxford University Press, Oxford

Walton, H.J. (1983) 'Individual Psychotherapy' in Kendell, R.E. and Zealley, A.K. (Eds) *Companion to Psychiatric Studies 3,* Churchill Livingstone, Edinburgh

Wing, J.K. Cooper, J.E. and Sartorius, N. (1975) *The Measurement and*

Classification of Psychiatric Symptoms, Cambridge University Press, Cambridge

Wolpe, J. (1958) *Psychotherapy by Reciprocal Inhibition*, Stanford University Press, Stanford

Yalom, I.D. (1983) *Inpatient Group Psychotherapy*, Basic Books, New York

Subject Index

typhoid fever 195

ulcerative colitis 116, 122
underweight 161
uraemia 165-6

vaginitis 158-9
veganism 123
venereophobia 172-3
verbal expression 35-6
violence 26, 46
visual evoked potentials 79
vocational assessment 13
vomiting 162-3

vulnerability 20

WAIS 258
water intoxication 237
weakness 210
Wernicke-Korsakoff syndrome
  90
WISC 258
withdrawal states 40
World Health Organization 99
writer's cramp 184

Yin and Yang 3

Author Index